HEALTH AND HAPPINESS FOR A LONGER LIFE

A guide to staying young

1st Edition

Tadeu Godoy

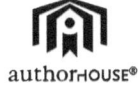

authorHOUSE®

AuthorHouse™ UK Ltd.
500 Avebury Boulevard
Central Milton Keynes, MK9 2BE
www.authorhouse.co.uk
Phone: 08001974150

First published by AuthorHouse   3/8/2011.

ISBN: 978-1-4567-2419-1 (sc)
ISBN: 978-1-4567-2420-7 (dj)

Front Cover: Elaboration and Art
Paulo Henrique Firmino
Front Cover Photos:
Ramires Fotografia e Vídeo and Osmar Rogieri
Portuguese Revision: Doctor Luiz Américo L. Nogueira
Translation: Patricia Cline Martins de Sá

Dear Reader,

My first job, at the age of 13, was in a pharmacy that belonged to a doctor, and which was located above his medical clinic.

This ten-year period of contact with the pharmacy, in which I assisted many patients, resulted in the birthing of an ardent desire in my heart to be a doctor, so that I could take care of people's health.

When I was about 32, I realized that my dream of going to medical school was not to become a reality. I then decided to write a book that would fulfill the role of a "health guide", that would be an instrument to help people enjoy perfect health, not only of the body, but also of the soul and spirit.

The reason for this approach is that I believe that the human being is a triune being. Also, many specialists in the area of psychology and parapsychology have confirmed that the majority of illnesses that affect humanity are psychosomatic in origin, and many are also caused by problems of the spiritual order.

After arriving at these conclusions, I intensified my studies in the areas of medicine that deal with both physical and psychological health, and on research that focuses on these themes.

Based on the studies and research of over 40 years, and on my own personal experience, and seeing that the methodology I have adopted has brought about excellent and incontestable results, I can affirm that it is possible to have perfect health and to prolong youthfulness and longevity.

In order for this to happen, one must simply follow certain criteria concerning care for the body, as well as certain principals and rules concerning care of the emotional and spiritual psyche.

My personal experience, and that of my wife, is the greatest proof that the methodology that we have adopted truly works, and produces notable, highly positive results.

In the photo on the cover, taken when I turned 60, one can observe that I had the appearance of someone 20 years younger. At this age, whenever I asked anyone how old they thought I was, the answer was always, "Oh, about 38, 40." The same thing happened when I was 40 years old – people would guess that I was 20 to 22. This can be seen in the sequence of photos – original and authentic - on the back cover of this book, taken when I was 20, 30, 40, 50, and 60.

However, the question of physical appearance is not the most important one. What is important is the fact that I have arrived at middle age, passing 60, with the same physical characteristics and appearance that I enjoyed in my 20's, with excellent energy and vitality.

My objective in writing this book is to provide a self-help tool, that will contribute towards more positive lives for people, so that they will be able to find the way to perfect health, as well as prolonged youthfulness and longevity, thus enjoying full, healthy, and happy lives.

The Author

Acknowledgments

I would like to express my sincere gratitude to my friends Dr. Artenio Olívio Richter, Dr. Adelmo Almeida de Oliveira, and Dr. Luiz Américo Limberti Nogueira for their support, encouragement and precious opinions.

Dr. Artenio is a plastic surgeon, scientist, researcher, and author, who earned his postgraduate specialization in Holland and in Germany. He is a member of the Brazilian Medical Society and the Brazilian Society of Mesotherapy. He developed his own method of dietetic counseling and weight control (weight loss). He also created a method for internal and external rejuvenation using cutaneous mesotherapy.

He is a highly knowledgeable student of ortho-molecular medicine (highly developed in the United States), and of modern methods of rejuvenation using oxygen, ozone, cell-therapy, thyme extract, serum therapy, procaine, enzymes, and combined proteins. He does research on the utilization of magnetic therapy and bio-energy in preventive medicine. He is also the creator of Body Clean, a technology and philosophy used exclusively in alternative treatments in curative medicine, which has highly positive results in the curing of various sicknesses.

Dr. Adelmo is a specialist in cardiology and circulatory system disease. He is a member of the Campinas Society of Medicine and Surgery, the Paulista Medical Association, the Brazilian Medical Association, the Brazilian Cardiology Association, and the Brazilian Eco-Cardiograph Society.

He concluded various courses in the area of cardiology and medical science, and has participated in numerous national and international congresses and symposiums. For many years he has fulfilled relevant functions at the Irmãos Penteado Hospital and at the Campinas Cardiology Institute in the State of São Paulo, which has made him one of the most respected cardiologists in the region of Campinas. He has presented works in congresses, and at the Medical Assembly of the State Servitor's Hospital in the city of Rio de Janeiro, which granted him an "Honorable Mention" diploma.

Dr. Luiz Américo Limberti is a specialist in colon proctology and diseases of the digestive tract. He worked many years as Assistant Professor of Surgery at the College of Medical Sciences of the Pontif Catholic University in Campinas.

I also want to thank Dr. Franz Salces Ruiz, PhD., who acquired his Chemical Engineer degree in Chile, and his post-graduate and doctorate degree in Nutritional Engineering at Unicamp, Campinas. I also extend my appreciation to Eliezer Pereira de Barros, theologian, philosopher, psychoanalyst, and writer; Neila Maria Schwartz, psychologist and pedagogue; José Paulo Val Costa, philosopher; and to Dr. Belmiro Targa, to Dra. Lorena Aguirre Zambrano Velho and Dra. Natália Aguirre L. Zambrano Barnes for their precious opinions and encouragement.

Contents

Preface

The issue of physical and mental health, of prolonging youth and longevity, is one of the most debated and discussed in the media. This is due to the tremendous importance that these factors represent for the life of a human being.

According to experts and researchers on the subject, for one to be able to enjoy good health, as well as find a way to a full and wholesome life, there are factors, basic rules, and principles that must be followed.

The fact that many people begin to suffer illness and to age prematurely is related to their lifestyles and to their behavior. Depending upon one's lifestyle and behavior, it is possible to break basic rules and ignore many principles.

As a result, we can see what statistics have shown us: people who, at a very young age, already suffer from diseases and illnesses that, historically, were found only in people over the age of 60. This has resulted in a regression of time in many lives. How many untold multitudes could have arrived at the age of 100, in perfect health, but instead died before the age of 60, simply for having lived an undisciplined lifestyle!

The main motive that allowed the author to reach the age he has, enjoying perfect health and discovering the way to a healthy and pleasurable life, is simply due to the fact that he adopted a correct life methodology, and has followed principles and basic rules that make this possible.

This fact has been a reality in his personal life experience because one day, when he was young, he made the decision to live a correct lifestyle, and adopted rules and principles that helped him to surpass middle age with a healthy and youthful body. He has also found the way to a harmonious and healthy life.

Enjoying good health and living a happy life are within the reach of any human being. But for this it is essential that one considers the body as the greatest patrimony that he possesses on this planet, and that he adopt a correct lifestyle.

There is a popular saying that goes like this: "It's never too late to start!" It never is too late to start something in this life, especially when dealing with health and happiness, for both health and happiness are factors that are within reach and at the disposition of anyone who wants them.

To obtain them, one only needs to use good sense and a little bit of intelligence; two extremely important qualities that the human being receives as an inheritance along with the precious gift called life.

Dr. Artenio Olivio Richter

Life is the Victory Prize

The formation of the human being, at the beginning of its life in its mother's womb, is something that transcends human intelligence. It can be considered a supernatural phenomenon, for it is a divine gift that all human beings had the privilege of receiving one day, according to the will of the Creator of the Universe.

The story of a human life has its beginning at that moment, when two seeds, attracted by a supernatural force, consummate the ritual of conception.

My story, since the day that my biological self began formation, is the same as all human beings. We were generated in the same way, and have the same similarities, both physical and emotional.

If this is true, why then do we not equally enjoy lives of abundant health, peace, joy, and happiness? Why is it that so many people are unable to achieve the peace and happiness to which we all have a right? My objective in narrating my story from the beginning is that, before I finish, all who read it will be able to open their minds to a new reality, and to see the light that signals the straight path to a healthy and happy life. My story, since its beginning, is the fantastic story of every human being.

A very long time ago – I don't remember when or where – I heard the voice of a great power saying to me, "You are going on a fantastic journey, where you will live incredible experiences in a land of wonders. There you will have every imaginable chance to enjoy a pleasurable life, as well as the opportunity to achieve another prize; that is, to live in yet another place called Paradise. But in order to go on this trip, you will have to compete in a big race, and there will be just one victor. Those who do not pass the finish line will not win the great prize."

Suddenly I heard something like an explosion, and there I was, running, running, running... All around me beings similar to myself were running desperately, trying to pass me. Several times many were able to. Time

1

accelerated and my strength began to wane. The groans of the competitors were deafening, and it was clear that there were millions of us.

Motivated by an ardent desire to go on this great journey, and aware that if I did not win, I would not live, a mysterious force pushed me onwards. And when I thought that I could go no further, there I was, nearing the finish line, the mark that would be the beginning of the great journey. I strained forward with all of my strength, until I broke through... I was embraced by something that received me warmly. It was my mother's egg. My soul quaked and my voice rang out, "I did it! I won! I am the champion!"

In this state of spirit, overcome by exhaustion, I don't remember whether I fainted or whether I slept. When I came back to consciousness, something extraordinary was happening. My body was being transformed. I could see my little feet forming into shapes, as well as the fingers on my hands. I rubbed my face and could sense that a great transformation had occurred in my body.

Time passed and I observed that my body continued being transformed, growing. Then at a certain point I saw a great brightness, and strange and huge beings all around me. I looked at my body and perceived that I looked like them.

I was afraid, and I remember that I cried a lot. Someone said, "It's a boy!", and everyone was smiling with joy. The miracle of life was consummated. The one whose egg had received me took me in her arms, and, smiling, said gently, "My dear son, welcome to life! Congratulations, Champion! You're the best, you're the victor! You are a victor at birth! I promise that I will do everything possible to make this fantastic voyage, called life, sublime and victorious until the end, until the day that the Creator calls you to give you the crown of glory."

This is a fictitious story about the beginning of life. But I am sure that it is not imaginary: I was, indeed, born a victor! Each one of us human beings is born a victor, for among millions of sperms we were the ones who won the race, had the great privilege of being conceived, and won the grand victory prize, called LIFE.

The Biological Limit of Life

Many researchers have proven that the human being is biologically able to live 120 years of age. And if it is possible to reach such an age, we could conclude, as well, that it should be probable that we reach at least 70 to 90% of this period with good health and vitality.

This means that, according to logic, we could easily arrive at the age of 80, 90, or even pass the age of 100 with healthy bodies. Reality, however, has shown that it isn't that simple, and proof of this is the very small number of people who reach the age of 90. Studies made by specialists show that there are various factors that contribute towards a person's being able to reach or surpass these age limits. Among them are having perfect health and a happy life.

For quite a long period of time I collected obituaries from a certain widely circulated newspaper, and discovered that the average age of death of older persons was between 70 and 80 years of age.

Although this data does not reflect scientifically attained statistical reality, it does show that most adults, upon reaching 50% of their biological potential (i.e. the age of 60), are already in a state of degenerative health, and therefore die prematurely.

The research that I have done over the years shows that the majority of people begin to present signs of aging in their 40's, and quite a few people even earlier. It is during this age range that the most common signs begin to appear: wrinkles, flaccidity of the skin and muscles, baldness, graying hair, weight gain, degenerative diseases such as circulatory, glandular, and hormonal disturbances, bone, hearing, and vision deficiencies, and the loss of vitality.

From the time I was a young teenager, I thought that youth - as it is one of the most beautiful and important phases in relation to physical appearance, health, energy, and vitality - should be longer. Youth begins in adolescence and lasts until about the age of 25 to 27, which is when, according to specialists, one's total physical structure is complete. It can last a few more years for some people, depending on their genetic makeup and other factors.

It was at this time in my youth that I began to try to think of a formula that would prolong youthful vitality. The reason for this is that my parents had a large number of siblings, and I, consequently, had a large number of cousins. I observed as these cousins grew and passed the age of 17, 19, 21 years of age, and older.

I noticed that from the age of 17 to 25, they had attractive bodies, and youthful beauty was evident in every aspect. The physical appearance of many of them, however, after passing the age of 25, began to change, due to weight gain and premature hair loss. Still others developed internal disturbances and illnesses. Others lost their sense of humor and joy, factors which, to a certain extent, dull joviality.

Observing these changes and transformations, I began to analyze the factors that make people seem older, and I developed an interest in learning about the human body, so that I could discover the factors that contribute towards maintaining youth, and those that accelerate the aging process.

After many years of observation, study, and research, and after understanding that the body is a complexity of matter, soul, and spirit, I came to the conclusion that any method, to be effective, must follow rules for the physical (body), the mental and emotional (soul), and the spiritual (spirit).

I believe that a person will only feel complete and fulfilled upon adequate nourishing of the physical body (with good and healthy things), the mind (with good and positive things), and the spirit (with divine attributes).

Based on my own personal experience, I can affirm that it is possible to retard the signs of aging and to live middle age (40 to 60 years of age) in perfect health, and with the same energy and vigor of the golden phase of youth, and that this is also possible after passing the age of 60.

The basic rules and methods that I have adopted are no great secrets, and can be practiced by anyone, regardless of their sex or age. It is logical, however, that the earlier one begins to practice such rules, the better the results will be in his future.

One of the great ills of humanity is that we tend to want to live for the intensity of the moment, with no regard for the consequences in the future. Therefore anything seems valid, even if the actions practiced are harmful to the body.

The same benefits that I have enjoyed as a result of meticulously following a correct lifestyle and life philosophy, which have brought positive results, can certainly be enjoyed by any person who is willing to do the same. For this, changes in mentality and behavior are necessary, and this will only be possible for those who truly value their lives and make living a better existence in this passing life a goal. All of us human beings are graced with the free will to choose that which will make our destinies sweet or sour, throughout the duration of, as well as at the end of, our individual stories.

To live well, to have a happy and healthy life, to prolong youth and life, depend exclusively upon each one of us. Any human being can enjoy an abundance of health, peace, joy, and happiness. All it takes is the use of good sense, and the good use of the free will that is given us by the Creator.

Longevity Depends on a Healthy and Happy Life

To live a healthy and happy life is the desire of every normal human being. And to prolong youth and life is also one of the main desires of the large majority of adults. This is evidenced by the fact that health and longevity are subjects that are widely addressed by the media. I believe that never before has there been such discussion about how to conserve health and youth as in our days. Science and Medicine have presented many theories as to the causes of the aging process. And, also thanks to Science and Medicine, today man has the hope of prolonging youth and increasing his life expectancy, as has been the case in many countries.

On the other hand, Science is alarmed at the growing number of premature deaths in recent decades, and at the diversity of illnesses that have contributed towards the decrease of life expectancy.

After studying and researching for years about the factors that contribute towards the retarding and the speeding up of the biological aging process, I was able to develop a methodology that made it possible for me to pass the age of 60, and yet conserve the same physical characteristics of when I was 25. That is, the same weight, minimal hair loss, healthy and wrinkle-free skin, firm muscles, and strong bones. Besides this, I also enjoy perfect health, excellent vitality and energy, and the appearance of someone 20 years my junior.

How many people have been able to surpass the age of 60, while conserving all of the physical characteristics of youth? I am sure that the number is very small. However, as this is a biological possibility, it should be a normal fact for the majority.

On my research spreadsheet, I have the names of dozens of relatives, friends, and acquaintances, with whom I maintain constant contact so that I can observe the physical and internal alterations which occur over time. I can confidently say that up until the present date I have never met anyone in my age bracket who has kept all the characteristics of their youth, and those who enjoy perfect health are very rare.

Those who maintained the same weight and hair had aged skin and gray hair. Those who had preserved their hair, skin, and youthful facial appearance, faced problems with their weight. The majority presented various diseases, such as hypertension, rheumatism, arthritis, diabetes, high levels of cholesterol and triglycerides, vascular insufficiency, organic, glandular, hormonal and nervous disturbances, accentuated loss of vitality, and other problems that affect health, contribute to the degeneration of the body, and anticipate aging.

In analyzing the opinions of specialists and researchers concerning the factors that contribute to the acceleration of the aging process, I discovered that the most frequently mentioned were: an erroneous life style, poor eating habits, a sedentary and undisciplined life, harmful vices, nervous system disturbances, stress, and inevitable diseases.

Based on my own studies and personal experience, I can affirm that the factors which bring about premature aging are numerous, and are related to individual behavior and LIFESTYLE. The factors that most contribute towards slowing down the aging process are: special care of the body, a diet that is balanced and rigorously controlled, regular physical exercise, a positive mind frame, emotional balance, self-control, mental exercise, and the cultivation of the spiritual man.

It was upon these factors that I based the method which I have meticulously followed, in order to live a healthy and happy life, and to reach the age I have, still maintaining youthfulness. If I had not adopted and followed a correct methodology since my youth, I am absolutely certain that today I would present a totally different state of health and physical appearance, and would appear much older than I do. That is, if I were even alive, for before deciding to radically change my way of living, I lived in a totally undisciplined manner.

Analysis of Lifestyle

Our lifestyle is related to our manner of living, and to all that we do and feel throughout each 24-hour period. The factors related to lifestyle that most influence our state of health are: the air we breathe, the water we drink, the foods we consume, our levels of stress, our physical activity, and our emotional state.

Any well informed person knows that, in our day, the air that we breathe cannot be considered of good quality, especially in the larger urban centers, where there is a large concentration of industry, vehicles, and smokers, which are the greatest contributors towards environmental pollution. There are cities and regions where the air that we breathe contains a high percentage of pollutants, soot, and toxic gases, highly harmful to the human organism and health.

Air – rather, the oxygen in the air we breathe, the primary element for sustaining human life - depends upon trees, plants, and forests. Scientists have shown that the solution for reverting the "greenhouse effect," which has been provoked by global warming, ever increasing in recent decades, is to plant millions of trees.

I cannot but manifest my indignation at the lack of conscience of the people who disregard and devalue nature. I find it tremendously absurd when I see someone destroying plant and animal life to substitute it with concrete, in simple carelessness. These people need to know that they are contributing towards the increase of air pollution, and the deterioration of the quality and purity of the oxygen that they themselves breathe, which will sooner or later influence their state of health and the period of time they will spend in this world.

Any well informed person is aware that the majority of the rivers that run through our cities have waters that are polluted and contaminated by chemical substances, heavy metals, and fecal coliforms, which are highly harmful to the human organism and health.

In the same manner that I am indignant concerning people's disregard for nature, by not concerning themselves about the deterioration of the quality of our air, I am also indignant concerning the lack of concern of those who pollute our sources of drinking water. Once I heard a phrase used by a group of ecologists: "If you don't love nature, leave her alone, for one day she will seek revenge!"

Another item that is, each passing day, becoming a greater and greater risk for the health of the world population is our diet. The industrialization of food is good in the sense that it makes life easier and provides more convenience. On the other hand, industrialized foods generally come with the addition of chemical additives such as preservatives, artificial coloring, flavoring, and other chemical substances, which, if consumed frequently and constantly, result in the accumulation of toxins in the organism. These toxins will most likely cause harm, and generate disturbances that will gradually provoke imbalance in the operational systems of the organism, which can lead to diverse illnesses for the body.

As an example, if we analyze industrialized chicken, we will find substances such as synthetic female hormones, which are utilized to accelerate the growth of the birds. This type of hormone, according to studies that have been released, may be responsible for several malefactors in the human organism, such as myoma (tumor that usually manifests in the muscular tissue), ovarian cysts, growth disturbances, hormonal and glandular disturbances, among others.

Even natural foods, such as fruits and vegetables, are largely contaminated by pesticides, insecticides, etc. These substances are harmful to the human organism, and if consumed frequently, certainly result in damage to the body, therefore affecting the state of health.

Therefore the air, the water, and the foods we consume are all carriers of toxins that accumulate in the body, and, over time, are responsible for innumerable ills that affect human health. For this reason many conscientious people are seeking a return to older customs, adopting healthier lifestyles, for they understand the value that air, water, a natural diet, and nature have for the life and health of the human race.

According to the naturalistic doctor, Dr. Artenio Olivio Richter, a high stress level is one of the main causes of the most common sicknesses that affect man at this current time in history. A person who is constantly under great stress usually presents nervous disturbances that cause health problems such as gastritis, gastric ulcers, and circulatory disturbances, which lead to greater and more serious sicknesses.

The more common symptoms of disturbances of nervous origin are: frayed nerves, constant nervousness, irritability, anxiety, insomnia, and depression. These can lead to digestive and intestinal disturbances, constipation, gastritis, gastric ulcers, renal deficiency, lumbar and sciatic pain, and others, which lead to more serious and harmful problems.

The lack of physical activity and exercise is a lifestyle factor of vital importance, which has tremendous repercussions on one's health, as we will see in the chapters on this subject.

As for emotional health, among the factors that can influence health are lack of adequate rest (which can generate serious disturbances for the nervous system, thus provoking imbalance in the other systems of the organism), and constant bad humor, the negative thoughts that oppress and affect the state of spirit. In following chapters I will deal with this subject in greater detail.

These are the main factors that constitute the lifestyle of each individual, and which determine whether or not we will live life in a full and healthy manner.

Analysis of the State of Health

During the many years that my professional activity was related to the area of preventive medicine, I often asked people the following question: "How is your health?" The two most common answers were "My health is fine!" or "My health is great!" After investigating and analyzing their state of health, however, I would come to the conclusion that these answers did not correspond to reality.

When I began to study about preventative health methods, I learned from great health professionals, such as Dr. James Scala, PhD, one of the greatest nutrition specialists in the world (and supervisor of the NASA nutrition program for astronauts), as well as from other preventive medicine experts such as Dr. Artenio Olivio Richter. From them I learned that the secret to perfect health lies in the harmonious balance among nine systems of the organism: the digestive, the intestinal, the circulatory, the urinary, the respiratory, the glandular, the nervous, the structural, and the immunological.

To evaluate one's state of health, one only needs to carefully verify how these nine systems are functioning, evaluating the symptoms and disturbances, signs which clearly indicate the state of health.

As an example, I will cite the case of a young lady, age 22, whose answer concerning her health was, "It's great!" After the evaluations, it was determined that her state of health was not as good as she had thought. The symptoms and disturbances recorded were the following: She had digestive difficulties, suffering from frequent heartburn and signs of gastritis. She had problems with constipation; she would go five or six days without a bowel movement. She suffered constant headaches. Her appetite was out of control, and she weighed 12 kilos above the weight considered proportional to her stature and bone structure. She suffered hair loss, dry skin, premenstrual cramps, insomnia, anxiety, and irritability. She suffered frequent back pain and physical debilitation.

By the irregularities noted in the evaluation, it was possible to conclude that the systems in her organism were not functioning harmoniously, and were unbalanced, especially the digestive, intestinal, glandular, structural, and nervous systems. Without changes in her lifestyle and improvements in her state of health, without a doubt, within a few years, she would fall victim to more serious disturbances and sicknesses.

Is it possible to do a self-analysis of one's own state of health? Yes! One only needs to observe the signs and symptoms manifest by the body. Headaches, for example, are a sign that there is some abnormality in the organism, which might be related to the digestive or nervous system, or can be the manifestation of a symptom of some sickness.

In order to determine whether or not there is an imbalance in the functioning of the organism systems, all one has to do is note the most common signs manifested by the body when an irregularity exists. The most common of these are: physical tiredness and overall debilitation; low resistance to disease; body odor or bad breath; frequent digestive problems; constipation; allergies; moodiness; nervousness and irritability; anxiety, stress, cramps, tingling and numbness in the arms and legs; back pain and sciatic nerve pain, joint pain, insomnia or excessive sleepiness; thin and fragile fingernails; excessive hair loss, faulty memory, bags under the eyes, chronic mucus in the nose and throat, etc. These are the signs and symptoms that are normally noted by preventive medicine or orthomolecular specialists in order to verify one's state of health.

To maintain balanced functioning of the nine organism systems, I follow some criteria and care. I use natural herbal and plant-based products as nutritional supplements, which contribute towards the balance of these systems. Periodically I use phyto-therapeutic products (made from plants), which remove toxins, cleanse, harmonize, and strengthen the nine systems of the organism.

When I turned 60, I could attest to the fact that my health was better than when I was 26. At that time, when I had my first assessment to evaluate my state of health, I suffered from digestive problems, gastritis, excessive gases (constipation), stomachaches (the beginning of an ulcer), and frequent throat and lung irritations.

However, at the age of 60, my state of health was excellent. This was corroborated by a series of medical and laboratory examinations that I undertook with the cardiologist Dr. Adelmo Almeida de Oliveira. The report showed the following results: "Excellent hemodynamic condition" ("hemodynamic" refers to the mechanics of the circulation of the blood;

"excellent condition" means that no negative factors exist which would interfere in the circulation).

It also included the results of the following examinations: Electrocardiogram, blood pressure, pulse, level of Glucose (blood sugar), Creatin, Urea, Potassium, Sodium, Triglycerides, and the three types of Cholesterol (LDL, HDL and Total). All the results were within normal ranges.

Besides these exams, I took some tests for the assessment of physical resistance, both pulmonary and cardiovascular. I rode a bicycle for two hours, with varying degrees of inclinations. After this I ran up a long flight of stairs, with no difficulty whatsoever, and without any abnormal reaction such as rapid heart beat or lack of air.

These exams confirmed that all of the systems in my organism were balanced and functioning in perfect harmony, resulting in an excellent state of health for someone my age. Besides this, I had not even suffered as much as a common cold for nearly ten years.

When I turned 62, I underwent a new series of cardiology, clinical, and laboratory exams, including a prostate exam. The results of the cardiology exams, and all of the laboratory exams were within normal ranges. Though these results were normal, chronic trauma to a vertebra in my backbone was detected, caused by two accidents that I have suffered. Unfortunately, this trauma to the vertebra interrupted a cycle of perfect health, as it is an irreversible and degenerative malady which will affect, in both the short and long term, my state of health. The way in which I deal with this will depend much upon my preparation, psychological balance, and spiritual maturity.

Knowing, Liking, and Caring for the Body

Learning about the body, in all of its facets, was my starting point. As easy as this may seem, it requires years of study and research. To illustrate how difficult it is to truly know the human body, I will use the example of medical doctors. They dedicate from 8 to 10 years to the study the body, and yet this period of time is insufficient for them to learn about a reality that surpasses human capacity, due to its complexity.

I consider the human body to be the most fantastic creation in the universe. I am so fascinated when I set out to investigate it, that sometimes I have the impression that I am traveling inside of it, contemplating the perfection of this magnificent work. Its engineering can only be the work of divine hands. I cannot understand people who, in their nearsightedness, do not perceive or believe that they were created by the powerful hands of a Creator. Nothing in this world was created without prior planning on someone's part. Therefore I understand that nothing on this immense planet that we inhabit appeared by chance.

Physiologically we have similar bodies, though there are many variations of physical appearance. Even though the organs and their functions are the same, the way they work, their reactions, and the behavior of the organism can vary. What is beneficial for some may not be for others. That is why it is so important that each one know his own body, and how it works, because in knowing its limits and reactions, it becomes easier to discern what is beneficial, and what is not.

For this it is necessary to have a good understanding of each organ, of each component, and of each element of the body. Once I asked a group of pre-university students about a certain component of the body and its specific function. Despite the fact that there were biomedical science students among them, no one could answer the question correctly. In another instance, when I emphasized the vital importance of water for the body, one student commented that he never drank much water, nor had he considered this to be an important factor.

In reality, all that makes up part of the constitution of the human body, such as water (which makes up about 80% of our organism), is fundamental, and fulfills specific functions. The purpose of this comment was to emphasize that most people do not know their own bodies.

There is still much indifference in relation to seeking information and knowledge, and methods for caring for the body, even though in recent years there has been an increased interest in the subject. I believe that this is due to the great attention that the media has given to stimulate physical culture and care of the body.

When I began to be interested in knowing more about my body, I would analyze and admire its complex structure. Thus my interest in studying the secrets of this "masterpiece" arose. This happened when I was growing up, and my physical structure was changing; I saw some details about my physical appearance that displeased me. Therefore I decided to begin a series of physical exercises in order to shape the parts that I did not like. And while I sought to improve my physical appearance, I also began to study "formulas" so that I could take care of my internal organs at the same time.

It is practically impossible to follow any method, with the objective of improving physical appearance, and especially internal functioning, without first acquiring knowledge about physiology and the factors that influence the state of health.

As for liking the body, this depends on the individual. I use the word "like," not in the sense of vanity, but to like the body for its intrinsic value. Unfortunately, due to the concepts of beauty that are imposed upon us, a beautiful and well-shaped body is thought of as being more valuable, while a less formed one is considered less valuable.

Not everyone has the privilege of having a perfectly sculptured body. There are an infinite number of factors that determine the physical type of each individual. Those who stand in front of the mirror and analyze their appearance will most likely find defects, or details that displease them. This was my case. Since I was very thin, I knew that it would not be very difficult to improve my physical appearance. All I needed to do was adopt an adequate diet and exercise program. Thus I began to exercise regularly, take greater care in terms of nutrition, and follow other important procedures.

When I began to serve in the military, over the age of 18, my body was more handsome and well-shaped than before. This influenced my state of mind and made me like myself better, due to the emotional satisfaction it brought. This is an important factor for inhibition, and for facilitating personal and social relationships.

Liking one's self and body, and considering one's worth, are fundamental prerequisites for human relationships and personal success. This I learned from personal experience, for before beginning the exercises I had some complexes and was timid and withdrawn.

Many people live their lives ill-at-ease, withdrawn, frustrated, and with complexes, simply because they are dissatisfied with their physical appearance and with themselves.

Frustration can lead to psychological problems, which can hinder a free and uninhibited life. In this case, the best medicine is to act, rather than to become indignant and full of self-pity. Self-deception never helps to solve problems; there is no one better than we ourselves to do something for ourselves. Therefore we have to decide what needs to be done in order to improve our situation, and then do it.

Esteeming the body is fundamental if there is to be interest in taking care of it. He who really likes his body should never attack it. He who loves his body esteems life. For those of you who do not like your bodies, I would say: First of all, remember the miracle of life. You are a champion! You won the precious gift of life to live it and to enjoy it. Don't allow the insignificance of the appearance of your body hinder you from enjoying what was given you. Look in the mirror and tell yourself, out loud, "I am a champion...I am a champion...I am a champion... I am a victor!" And begin to live like one.

Also, a person's beauty is not confined to his exterior; what brings out beauty comes from the inside – the nobility of character and of spirit. What truly distinguishes the beauty of a person are virtues such as humility, kindness, cordiality, and moderation of behavior and communication. Many would-be beautiful people have an unpleasant appearance because their interior is horrible. To want to is to be able to. The one, who desires to change, certainly can. Therefore, for those who desire to see changes in their bodies or in their personality, now is always the time to start.

There are no ugly people, even those who are ill humored and bitter, or who have undesirable physical shapes. Everyone, without exception, has some beauty, regardless of manner, temperament, or individual style, for each of us is very important, especially to the One who created us. Each human being contributes towards the beautification of this planet on which we live.

After learning about the body and realizing the importance of health for a full life, we begin loving it and caring for it as a matter of natural course. As a result of this new focus, many diseases will be prevented, people will be much healthier, and, without a doubt, youthfulness and life will be prolonged for many additional years.

Taking Care of the Body

I have already stated that in order to take care of the body, it is necessary to be familiar with its entire physiology. This requires years of study and information about the organ, circulatory and respiratory systems, and especially about the autonomous nervous system and the endocrine, or glandular, system, for these are the ones that basically command the others.

Care for the body should, ideally, begin during the growing phase, but one can obtain good results even if he begins later.

There are many people who never worry about taking care of their bodies until the day that they are surprised to discover some sort of abnormality. They live undisciplined lives until, suddenly, they survive some unexpected malady, and generally the thought, "Whoa, I need to take care of myself!" comes to mind. The unexpected malady may be the announcement of a sickness that has installed itself in order to disrupt good health and bring about various troubles.

He who intends to take care of his body must begin doing so with certain unavoidable principles firmly planted in his mind: strength of will, dedication, and perseverance. There is very little benefit to be derived from exercising or following a diet for a while, then afterwards quitting.

It is also a good idea to undergo a physical evaluation. When I began taking care of my body I underwent several medical and laboratory exams. Since the results indicated some irregularities, my first step was to correct that which was out of order.

The results of this checkup revealed gastrointestinal disturbances, pancreatic deficiency, poorly functioning intestines (constipation), abnormal levels of uric acid, excessive blood sugar, the presence of crystals in the urine, and a common intestinal parasite.

These irregularities were the result of economic and familiar problems that I faced between the ages of 13 and 21, a very difficult phase that brought about turmoil of a physiological nature, as well as affecting the organs. During this phase of financial difficulty, I was unable to maintain a correct and healthy diet, which is the main factor for maintaining good health.

When things began to improve, all I had to do was follow a healthy diet, with the use of natural products and some special cares. This resulted in all of the stabilization of all the functions of my organism in less than a year, which was proven by a new round of medical exams.

Right now I can say that my health today is better than at the time I decided to start being more careful, because at the present time I suffer no irregularities, as evidenced in the last medical and laboratory exams I underwent, when I turned 64 (with the exception of the aforementioned spinal trauma).

Before discussing the special cares I have taken over the years, I need to clarify two points. First, I cannot describe them in detail, because not everything that is good and adequate for me will be good and adequate for everyone. I cannot intend that this book be a manual for perfect health. Second, since we are also made up of soul and spirit, I believe that there must be integration of body, soul, and spirit. Therefore it is necessary to simultaneously observe rules and principles in regard to the soul and spirit, as well as to the body.

In my opinion, man is only complete when there is harmony between the body, soul, and spirit. Without this, he will never achieve the balance and degree of maturity that are indispensable for mental and spiritual perfection, which, in turn, will provide a life of pleasure, joy, and happiness. These are necessary for a healthy life.

When I stated that a change of mentality is necessary, I was referring to this awareness that we must have that we are not mere matter, but that we also have a soul and spirit. Some may question this, but this affirmation has already been proven by studies made in the area of paranormality.

Many people fail to recognize the divine aspect of their nature because they do not believe that they were created by a supreme being. As a result they go through life in a mediocre dimension, unaware of the privileges that God prepared for His creation, at a much higher dimension – much higher than people can imagine.

The Bible promises us this: *"As the heavens are higher than the earth, so are my ways higher than your ways, and my thoughts than your thoughts"* (Isaiah 55:9). Also: *"No eye has seen, no ear has heard, no mind has conceived what God has prepared for those who love him"* (1 Corinthians 2:9).

When all human beings discover their divine nature, and the value hidden within it, sickness, mediocrity, imperfections, and the biological limit to life – which can well surpass 120 years - will all disappear. But as long as there are so many people who do not believe in, or ignore the existence of, their spiritual part, thus despising the teachings of the Creator, and neglecting due care of their greatest patrimony, their bodies, there will be sickness, suffering, destitution, and many elderly young people being buffeted by life.

Basic Care for a Healthy Body

External Parts:

Posture: The posture of the body is the most important point when it comes to personal physical appearance. It can make one more elegant or less elegant, more attractive or less attractive. Most people do not pay much attention to their posture, but good posture is fundamental for avoiding problems that naturally occur as the years go by. Spinal problems are among the greatest maladies that health specialists try to solve. Many people suffer back problems simply because they did not pay due attention to correct posture.

Correcting my posture, whether standing, sitting, or lying down, was one of the first steps I took. I learned to maintain correct posture even as I was seeking information to begin the series of exercises for the improvement of my physical aspect. Many people, even while still young, have the habit of maintaining an incorrect, even awkward, posture. This is why there are so many young people who already suffer from degenerative spinal problems.

I suggest that those who desire more information on the subject seek out books written by well-known specialists, who can provide more information.

Hair: From childhood I have enjoyed keeping my hair neat. I always showered it much care and attention. My genetic traits tend more towards the physical traits of my mother's side of the family. My relatives on her side, including cousins, nieces and nephews, for the most part have the problem of receding hairlines. Many of my cousins, soon after passing age 22, already began premature hair loss, and accentuated hair loss before the age of 30.

Up until the age of 50 I had no difficulty in maintaining a voluminous head of hair, but at that point I began losing quite a bit. The typical corners of the forehead, at the hairline, began increasing. I began taking special cares and intensified my massages, which I had already been doing for years. Thus I was able to maintain my hair volume.

The method that I use is effective. When I interrupt it, as a sort of test, I can tell a definite difference. I wash my hair once every two days, using a neutral shampoo followed by a natural, plant and herb based conditioner. For hydration I apply aloe vera oil and a composition of keratin; every 15 days I use an ampoule of Vitamin E, massaging it in with my fingers to stimulate circulation. I get a haircut every two weeks.

Facial skin: This is the most visible part of the body, and as it is most exposed to the elements, it is also the most damaged. It can be harmed by the sun, the cold, the wind, by pollution, or by internal factors such as the food consumed, disturbances of the organs, and disease. Maintaining good and healthy skin depends on various factors.

The most important factor is food intake. The second is how the organs are functioning. The third is the condition of the blood vessels in the facial region, it's oiliness, and moisture. Since the face is one of the places where signs of aging first appear, those who would like to retain their youthful appearance must take care of their faces from adolescence; the earlier the better. And we need to begin with the key factor: nutrition.

I attribute the good quality of my skin to the following factors: an adequate and healthy diet, which is rigorously controlled and based on natural products; adequate rest; special care to maintain the organism functioning perfectly, especially the digestive and urinary systems; regular exercise and massages; and periodic facial cleansing.

I use neutral soap. Since my skin is the dry type, I have been using daily, since age 45, a vegetable-based moisturizing lotion, enriched with vitamins A, E, and O3, which improves oxygenation, moisturizes, nourishes, and tones the skin, thus retarding signs of aging. In cold weather, when the skin is dryer, I increase my consumption of products rich in vitamins A, D, and E, such as cod liver oil, wheat germ oil and beer yeast.

Another factor of vital importance in maintaining good skin quality is the amount of water consumed during the day. I have always had the habit of drinking an average of two liters per day. Water influences the moisture, which is essential for maintaining the flexibility and elasticity of the skin.

Upon waking up, and upon lying down at night, I do facial exercises, which contribute towards keeping the facial muscles firm. If you would like to know more about these exercises, you can find such information in pamphlets and videos provided at aesthetic and plastic surgery clinics.

Forehead: The forehead is one of the first places where wrinkles begin to appear. Many people naturally have the habit of wrinkling the muscles of the forehead, without thinking about it or seeing it as a vice. While young, the skin is moist, oily, and flexible, so wrinkles do not appear. But, as the years pass, depending on the type of skin, even before the age of 30 wrinkles may already become well defined.

I have seen young people, barely over the age of 20, who already have deep wrinkles on the forehead. Normally this happens because they have the habit of contracting these muscles while talking, or when worried or depressed. I used to wrinkle my forehead, but when, at about age 35, I noticed that it was causing wrinkles, I trained myself to not do this. I also began special exercises and massages. As a result of this care I was able to keep the wrinkles from becoming more pronounced.

Eyes: The corners of the eyes are among the places where wrinkles appear very early on. The wrinkles in the outer corners, called crows' feet, begin to form due to constant contractions, especially when the skin is dry. Just like in the case of the forehead, many people have the habit of contracting the eye muscles without noticing it. Sometimes it is just a bad habit, and sometimes it is because the person dislikes bright light, or has poor vision, or it can even be for emotional reasons.

The care that I take to avoid wrinkles in this region are the following: I avoid contracting these muscles under any circumstance, save to smile. A normal smile contributes very little towards accentuating these wrinkles. In the event of excessive brightness, I use dark glasses with a good quality lens. Also, the series of facial exercises that I have adopted includes exercises that compensate and firm the muscles around the eyes.

Mouth: This is another point that is among the most visible, and one that influences a youthful appearance. Many people, after the age of 40, or even earlier, have the habit of biting on their lips as if they were sucking inwards. Some do it with the upper lip, some with the lower, and some with both. This helps to deform the shape of the mouth, as well as to decrease its fullness, thus diminishing its youthful appearance. Facial exercises help to maintain youthful appearance.

Neck: This is another of the most visible places where the first signs of aging can become apparent. There is an important detail that contributes towards many people appearing older than they are: it is their posture. In my studies I was able to prove that very few people pay attention to this fact, especially after the age of 30.

Since the head is one of the relatively heavy parts of the body, as time goes by, the neck tends to become more rigid. This makes the skin more flaccid, and helps the neck to become thicker and form a double chin, which, besides deforming, also causes wrinkles in the skin. Muscle and nerves are part of the support system of the neck, so I developed some specific exercises for stretching the neck and maintaining firm muscles.

The basis of these exercises are upward, downward, lateral, and circular motions. One only needs to stretch out the neck, and make these motions slowly and gently, repeating each one 5 times. I do these exercises before I go to sleep, because they serve to relax muscular tension. Another factor that contributes towards the formation of double chins and neck wrinkles is sleeping on a pillow that is too high, and the posture of the neck while sleeping.

Jaw: This is also a very visible area that can easily present deformities, mainly in people who are ill humored and habitually clinch their teeth. The chin needs care. I try not to clench my teeth or be ill humored. I frequently massage it with circular movements using the palm of my hand. Facial exercises also help avoid flaccidity of the jaw muscles and skin.

Armpits: Taking care of this part is important in order to prevent underarm odor, irritations, and infections caused by germs. I wash my armpits every day when I take a shower - more often, if needed - and I use a deodorant with a low alcohol content.

Chest and Thorax: These are important for one's physical and personal appearance, and are of the regions most perceivable to others. As I have the habit of doing specific exercises for this region, I have been able to keep these muscles firm, contributing to a more youthful appearance.

Abdomen: Firm abdominal muscles are very important in order to prevent "pot bellies." Since this is something that makes people look older, I do specific exercises for this area. The most practical exercise, and the one that brings about the best results, it the practice of breathing in deeply, with the stomach muscles tightened.

Backbone: It may not seem like it, but the spine plays a very important role, not only as the main support for the body, but also as one of the principal factors in maintaining a beautiful, elegant and youthful appearance.

Incorrect posture is the principal cause of diseases in the spine that occur in old age. The firmness of abdominal and back muscles is very important for correct posture and support of the body. Therefore flexing exercises that strengthen the muscles of the back and abdomen are essential.

Posture while sleeping: This is another important factor, not only for sleeping well and preventing spinal problems, but also in order to avoid face and neck wrinkles. Some specialists recommend lying on the side with the knees bent, especially for those who are overweight. I sleep on my back and very rarely on my side. In the health courses I have participated in, I have learned that the best position is on the back, for it facilitates the circulation of the blood for those whose weight is proportional to their height, and it also provides better muscle relaxation.

As for mattresses, the opinions of specialists vary considerably. It should have a firm base, and the firmness of support that is appropriate for each body structure type. I base my opinion on the fact that the first human beings slept on firm ground. My mattress is made up of one layer of undulated rigid plastic foam that is four inches thick. It is a special, anti-transpiration foam. The lower layer is made up of medium density foam, five centimeters thick. I use pillows of different thicknesses; one, two centimeters thick, when I sleep on my back, and another, twelve centimeters thick, when I sleep on my side.

Private Parts: When I worked in the drugstore, every day people came in to buy medicine for fungus and anal itches. For good personal hygiene, I recommend douching the anus after going to the toilet, using medicinal soap, and drying the area with a cotton towel. Besides being more hygienic, this also helps to prevent maladies like prurient anal itches and rashes that could lead to greater problems.

Hands: Many people do not realize that they frequently touch contaminated things. We are accustomed to itching our noses, rubbing our eyes and ears, etc. We frequently touch our mouth. Many diseases are transmitted via the hands. I wash mine several times a day, and try to pay attention as to the things and places I touch. The hands are also places where aging becomes apparent at an early age. Every day I moisturize them with the same lotion I use on my face and neck. Every week I cut and groom my nails and cuticles.

Feet: Foot problems are very uncomfortable. Working at the drugstore, I saw many people looking for medicine and advice about foot care. The most common problems are eczema, fungus, ingrown nails, corns, and bunions.

To avoid eczema and fungus, every day I wash and then carefully dry my feet, especially between the toes, and I always use clean socks. I also avoid using vulcanized or synthetic shoes. To prevent corns and calluses, I always buy well fitting shoes. Every week I cut my toenails to avoid ingrown nails.

Clothing: This is important for good health and for enhancing one's appearance. Clothes should always be kept clean, for they can retain and allow for the spread of germs and bacteria. Unfortunately we live in a society that measures the value of a person by his clothing, which is absurd.

Simple changes in the ways one dresses, such as fixing up the hair or taking care of the skin, can greatly help to change his appearance and his sense of well being, and also make him a more attractive and jovial person.

Internal parts:

I would like to be able to describe in greater detail all of the care and methods I use to take care of my internal parts, but I will do so only for the most important ones. The reason for this is that some could try to do what I do, but not obtain the same results. Each organism reacts in different ways, and each person is unique.

When I had pneumonia, I used natural products as medications, and my problem was resolved. However, a different person may have the same sickness, use the same products, yet have less favorable results.

Also, those who have diabetes or excessive uric acid are unable to use the products that I use. It is necessary to analyze each case, and its own set of deficiencies. If I were to mention many of the successful experiences that I have had, I would create controversy. Many health specialists do not believe in naturalistic medicine, nor do they support alternative medicines.

Teeth: The teeth are also a very visible part of the body. Nothing makes a person's presence more outstanding than a big and natural smile. It is also one of the principal characteristics of young, healthy people. A young person who rarely smiles is one who most certainly has some type of problem.

A pretty smile does not depend on a certain kind of teeth. But the teeth do need to be healthy, clean, and well cared for. Smiling is not difficult, and is good for the health. In order to always be smiling, and to have a happy semblance, one only needs to practice and make it a habit.

Throat: Before the age of 30 I suffered from frequent throat irritations, but this has happened very little since that age. When it does, I apply Do-

In touches at specific points, and use natural anti-inflammatory phyto-therapeutic products.

Respiratory System: Normally those who regularly practice sports and eat correctly have healthy lungs. I consider the lungs to be the most important organ in the body, for no one can survive more than 3 to 5 minutes without breathing. Therefore this organ needs special care.

I had bronchial pneumonia when I was a teenager, and again at the age of 47 (low resistance due to stress). After the sickness I underwent treatment using phyto-therapeutic products as expectorants and for cleansing, and adopted vitamin supplements to strengthen the lungs and the immunological system.

Digestive System: The digestive system is the first stage of food processing. Therefore, it must function perfectly, so that the second stage can also function perfectly. One who maintains a balanced and adequate diet is already practicing the fundamental care for the preservation and health of the organs contained in the digestive system: the esophagus, stomach, liver, pancreas, supra-renal glands, intestines, kidneys, and bladder.

When the digestive system works well, the heart, the circulatory system, the endocrine system and others, also work well. In short, a well regulated system is less subject to disease and is more resistant to sickness.

Intestinal System: My parents and grandparents always said that well functioning intestines avoid many a trouble, and that health and the quality of skin also depend on this. Today, according to my experience, I can affirm that this is true, and many specialists agree with me.

At the time I underwent my first exams to evaluate my state of health; one of the irregularities found by the doctor was poorly functioning intestines. Sometimes I would go three or four days without a bowel movement. Beside this, I also had the problem of excessive gases. I eliminated these deficiencies by adopting a diet that included natural products rich in fibers. Today my intestinal system functions with the regularity of clockwork.

According to specialists, one needs to have a bowel movement at least once a day, depending on the quantity of food consumed. Well functioning intestines contribute towards good and healthy skin, as well as a better balance of bacterial flora.

Urinary System: As the kidneys and bladder perform very important diuretic functions and the elimination of impurities, they also demand some special care. In the same way that an adequate diet benefits the digestive and intestinal systems, it also benefits the kidneys and bladder.

What most influences the proper functioning of the kidneys is the quantity of liquids consumed throughout the day. I customarily observe the density, color, and odor of the urine. When I feel that it is necessary, I use a 100% natural phyto-therapeutic product that works as a diuretic, and helps to eliminate impurities and prevent inflammations in the ureters, bladder, and urethra.

I could write many pages about care for the body, but I believe that this summary is sufficient to make people think more seriously about the subject. A simple disturbance in the digestive or intestinal system can, over time, bring about other disturbances in the organism, and ultimately become a serious illness.

Any and all care taken of the body, besides being important for short-term health, will most certainly result in positive results for a healthy future.

Exercise: An Indispensable Factor for Those who Value the Body

Exercise is indispensable for taking care of the body. As I sought more information about the benefits of regular exercise, I learned from cardiologists, lung specialists, orthopedists, and psychiatrists that exercise is of vital importance for keeping healthy and young. Unfortunately, a great many people do not know this.

And due to the fact that exercise is so indispensable for good health, keeping in shape, and preserving youth, I am going to discuss the modalities that I have practiced and comment about their effects.

What I have most enjoyed, since childhood, is walking. I usually walk three or four kilometers a day. I take large, vigorous, and rapid steps. For best results, walking should be fast enough to make the body sweat. It is a type of exercise that involves the muscles in general, and, because it demands more air and activates the circulation, it oxygenates the lungs and heart, thus improving the capacity of these organs.

I like to swim. Some psychologists say that swimming is excellent for the muscles and nerves. It is a sport that uses the whole body. Lung specialists consider swimming to be very good therapy for respiratory dysfunctions and for increasing pulmonary resistance.

Another sport that I also practiced for many years was rowing. It is one of the most complete exercises because it, too, involves all of the body. It strengthens the legs and shapes the thighs, as well as increases the biceps, triceps, back, and chest muscles. It tightens the stomach region due to the exertion of great force, especially in the legs.

I also ride a bicycle. I used to take long rides with a group of friends. I always completed the course and was among the first to finish.

I tried jogging, but it was never my favorite. Nowadays, when I run, it is never for more than five-hundred meters. I do this only to test my cardio-respiratory resistance. It is a good sport, but it is very demanding of the circulatory system, especially after age 40. For those who like to run, it is advisable to see a doctor for proper orientation to avoid complications.

I have always practiced the art of self-defense, and enjoy it very much. It strengthens the muscles, increases their flexibility and suppleness, improves one's sense of balance, dexterity and self-control, and speeds up the reflexes. It is disinhibiting and helps to control emotional reactions. This is a very salutary sport for both mind and body.

Another exercise that I like to do from time to time is pull-ups on a horizontal bar. This is recommended for strengthening the arm, chest, and abdominal muscles, and to improve one's overall appearance.

Although I had practiced intense physical activities since childhood, I only began to do regular exercises as a young man. From that time on I only interrupted practicing sports periodically, for six to eight months at a time, in order to verify the changes happening in my body.

Based on experiences I have had with sports in general, I am convinced that if I had not done these exercises regularly, I would not have the well-shaped body I have today, nor would I have kept the same appearance I had when I was 25. I would not be enjoying perfect health, abundant energy, and vitality, nor would I have kept this jovial appearance, even after the age of 64.

All sports should be practiced conscientiously, and with orientation and preparation. Whatever your age may be, I recommend that you talk to a doctor or physical trainer about an exercise and sports program that is suitable for you.

Exercise can be beneficial, but it can also cause future problems. It has been proven that, depending on the type or criteria adopted in exercising when one is growing up, exercise can cause growth and development problems, such as muscular diseases and back problems.

In conclusion I want to emphasize that although I have always played various sports and done exercises, I have never spent more than an hour a day in such activity. I always tried to alternate the types, and limited this activity to three times a week at most, which, according to specialists, is ideal.

Do Idleness and Inactivity Speed up the Aging Process?

All research concerning longevity indicates that idleness is one of the primary factors responsible for premature aging. There are two types of idleness. One is the lazy person, who dislikes any type of physical effort. This person cannot be considered healthy because usually his strength of will is totally dysfunctional. Disposition of spirit, ambition, and other factors that are indispensable for a pleasurable life are inhibited in him. Idleness can bring a person down to such a low level of complacency that he loses interest in any physical, or even mental activity.

The second type of idle person is one who is idle due to his circumstances, such as those who have sedentary work habits, or those whose work demands very little physical activity.

Geriatric specialists have proven that after the age of 40 certain changes begin taking place in the body, such as stiffness of the muscles responsible for posture, loss of agility, a slowing of reflexes, weakening of the muscles, physical debilitation, and flaccidity of the skin.

Knowing this I began observing people over 40 who were part of my daily life. After several years of observation I came to the conclusion that those who were idle suffered these alterations more rapidly and with greater intensity. When I worked in the area of health care, I accompanied several cases of people with chronic rheumatism, stiff muscles, and agility deficiency. All of these people had lived sedentary lives for years.

When I worked as a personal defense instructor, I had the opportunity to accompany the very interesting case of a person with atrophied muscles. This man, a 48-year-old Spaniard, came to me one day saying that he had a serious problem. He said that his muscles were stiffening, and that gradually he had been losing his flexibility and agility. He came to see me after watching one of my classes, and seeing that the exercises I taught the students were for elasticity and flexibility. He wanted to know whether or not I could help him.

After analyzing the case and verifying what type of treatment he was undergoing, and had undergone, I decided to accept him as a student. As his situation was somewhat delicate, besides the normal series of exercises that I normally assigned to my students, I added some specifically for stretching the strained back muscles.

In the beginning it was very difficult. I had to give him special attention and help him get through the series of exercises. It required much patience, for he had difficulty in maintaining balance and movements, especially in attack and defense moves.

By the third month, however, the results were good and noticeable. Since he was a dedicated and persistent student, by the sixth month he was able to keep up with the other students, most of which were under the age of 30. After a year of dedication, I had the pleasure of seeing him graduate as one of the best students in his class. It is very gratifying to see a person who once hobbled, with his head down and inhibited, be transformed into a recuperated, uninhibited, happy, and satisfied person. That is why I affirm that physical exercise can truly bring about miracles.

I have met many people who, though still young, are always discouraged, and even debilitated, because they lead idle lifestyles. It is common to find among young people those who have no motivation, no prospects, and who are totally disinterested in life. Many are depressed and begin having neurotic problems, simply because they do not occupy their minds or practice any physical or recreational activity.

For a period of time I worked with drug addicted youth, and I noticed that many gave themselves over to drugs out of boredom, as they had no occupation, nor did they have physical or mental activity. In the days in which we live, due to the variety of comforts that this world offers, it is a far too common thing to see a large number of people automatically succumb to idleness.

With automation, the use of the motor vehicles, and the decentralization of transportation, many get used to convenience without noticing that they are falling into idleness. Over time, after becoming conditioned by convenience, even a trip to a nearby supermarket is made by car, rather than on foot. This is one of the reasons that we see so many people today, even young people, suffering from rheumatism, circulatory disturbances, varicose veins, lack of resistance and vitality, and other symptoms more appropriate for those of an advanced age.

Those who have a sedentary lifestyle should develop an awareness of the value and necessity of exercise and regular physical activity, especially during the hours they are not working. The excuses of no time, a busy life, and day-to-day difficulties have led many people to fall into idleness. The main culprit is not a lack of time, but disinterest, apathy, and the desire for comfort.

Many evils could be prevented or delayed if there were more dedication and interest in physical activity and exercise. We can conclude then, from what has been said, that idleness does promote ageing and sickness. But, as the old saying goes, "It's never too late to start!"

In 1990 I watched a news report about the three oldest people in the country; one 98, one 113, and one 116. In the interviews, all three attested to the fact that one of the factors that contributed towards their longevity was physical activity. All of the studies about longevity that I have read agree that people who live past age 90 always have diverse and constant activities that provide intense exercise for the body.

Does Exercising Help Maintain Youth?

Many people, even those who do not regularly practice sports, spend a great deal of energy because of their occupations. This is the case of field workers and laborers. Studies made on these people indicate that they not only enjoy better health and physical resistance, but that they also maintain youthfulness longer. Other people of the same age, who also eat similar diets, but are less active, are considerably different.

Many businesses have sports associations in order to promote leisure and recreation, and to stimulate interpersonal and social relationships. But the main objective is to encourage the employee to exercise. The employee who exercises regularly enjoys better health and vitality, has better disposition and resistance, and is more productive. This has been proven in studies made by specialists.

Despite all of the publicity about the benefits of physical exercise for health, there is still a tremendous disinterest in actually practicing it. And this is quite a shame! Those who would practice exercise regularly would enjoy much better and healthier lives. Studies show that the large majority of cardiac patients between the ages of 30 and 50 never had the habit of regular physical activity.

Why is exercise so vital to our health? When we exercise our muscles they are naturally heated. With the activation of muscular fiber and the heating of the body, the circulation of the blood improves, thus benefiting the entire organism. This heating provokes sweating, which eliminates impurities from the body and disobstructs the skin pores. With the increase of the volume of air taken in by the lungs - which naturally occurs with exercise – and with the activation of circulation, the blood is enriched with more oxygen and other nutrients, which will nourish the cells and tissues. As he pores are decongested by transpiration, and the skin receives more nutrients, the epidermis - the non-venous surface layer - receives more moisture and oiliness, which are important factors for elasticity and a youthful and healthy appearance.

Exercise contributes towards strengthening the muscular fiber of the heart, and also towards the dilation of the cavities, thus increasing the quantity of blood pumped with each contraction. This decreases the number of heart beats, which facilitates and improves the work of the heart. In other words, it saves the heart excess work, thus decreasing the possibilities of cardiac deficiencies.

The lungs are benefited because during the exercises the blood passes through them faster. As the volume of air inhaled increases during the exercise, the veins dilate, thus increasing the area through which the oxygen passes into the bloodstream. Thus the thorax, the diaphragm, and the muscles are strengthened, and the efficiency of the lungs is improved, as well as their resistance.

The nerves, which are responsible for the activation of muscular fiber, are benefited and become more efficient in the transmission of electrochemical impulses and in the activation of muscular fiber, which result in resistance and physical strength.

The media frequently reports on positive results obtained by patients in psychiatric hospitals, resulting from the practice of regular physical exercise. It has been proven that the patients sleep better, consume less medication, and feel less anxiety. Besides all of the benefits that exercise provides for the body and mind, it is worth mentioning its outstanding effect on emotional balance and the state of spirit.

Since I have always attended clubs, sports gyms and academies, I have noticed something that is very common in these places. When people are talking, I always hear about the happiness and sense of well-being that exercise causes them.

Between 1977 and 1978 I was a personal defense instructor at ACM in Sao Paulo, one of the largest sports associations in the capital. There I also practiced weight lifting, gymnastics, and swimming. I worked on the night shift, when the sports arenas were extremely busy. During this period of time I was able to observe some important facts. I had students who used depressants, but after just a few weeks of regular exercise, would abandon the use of such medications, as problems with anxiety and insomnia would disappear.

I had the opportunity to meet several people who suffered from circulatory disturbances, who, at their doctor's orders, began to exercise. After a few months, under medical supervision, they abandoned their medications and the disturbances disappeared.

These facts convinced me, once for all, that physical exercise can bring about true miracles, as well as help solve problems of a psychological and emotional nature.

As I have always practiced exercises, I can affirm that they have provided me with all of the benefits I have mentioned, and have contributed towards firm muscles in general, which prevents muscular flaccidity. It has also firmed skin in the areas that normally give away a person's age.

Every five years, for my records, I have pictures taken of myself wearing the same shorts that I have kept for many years. Comparison of the pictures taken at age 20, 30, 40, 50, 60, and the most recent, at 62, proves that my body (physical type) is exactly the same, and maintains the same appearance of age 25. There have been no visible alterations, and I have maintained the same weight (65 kilos).

The Importance of Exercise For Health and Physical Vigor

Studies have proven that one of the symptoms of the degeneration of the body is the loss of physical vigor. Geriatrics and gerontologists confirm that those who exercise regularly have more vigor and vitality, as well as better health.

When I began to exercise regularly, I underwent some tests to evaluate my physical strength, pulmonary resistance, and cardiovascular capacity. After a year of practicing various modalities regularly, I underwent the same exams, and the results were surprising.

The things that had changed were the things that I had disliked about myself. Before, I was slightly hunchbacked, my chest looked "caved in," my arms were very thin, my thighs were curved almost 3 centimeters, I weighed 56 kilos, my height was 1.67 meters, my shoulders were curved inwards, and my overall physical appearance was thin, unkempt, and inelegant.

Afterwards my physical strength and pulmonary resistance doubled. My shoulders were straight, the measurement of my chest muscles increased almost 20 centimeters, my arm muscles increased, making them more attractive, my thigh muscles increased, and the curved in part disappeared. My weight went to 65 kilos, and my height to 1.7 meters. All of these changes resulted in a more handsome and elegant appearance.

This transformation brought about much personal satisfaction, which resulted in physical and mental well-being, thus improving my self-esteem.

I had this type of experience various times, by stopping the practice of exercise, as a test, and then restarting. I became convinced that good physical vigor depends upon regular physical exercise, as well as correct eating habits, vitamin supplements, adequate rest, and good mental disposition.

It has already been confirmed that the lack of physical exercise is among the main factors that lead to circulatory problems. Circulatory deficiencies caused by physical inactivity debilitate the muscles and nerves, and eventually affect physical vigor.

When I interrupted my exercise routine for several months, as a test, I noticed the following changes: my muscles diminished, as did my strength, vigor, and pulmonary resistance. I became more flaccid, my appetite was altered, I became restless and irritable, had more difficulty sleeping, and less physical disposition. This proves the great importance of exercise in order to maintain health and physical vigor.

Concepts of Health and Vitality

Health is defined as a state of fullness and normality of organ function. Some say that health is having energy, disposition, joy, and a good state of spirit, even in the face of illness. The World Health Organization defines health as the absence of sickness, and complete physical, mental, and social well-being.

In order to have good vitality it is essential to have good health. Vitality, or vital strength, should be a normal characteristic of those who have good health.

I define perfect health as having proportional balance between structure and weight, regular functioning of the internal organs, with no abnormalities, good immunological defense, balance of the automatic and motor nerves, good circulation, harmonious balance between the emotional psyche and spiritual satisfaction, good disposition, vigor, and enthusiasm, and the joy and pleasure of living.

My own personal experience is a rare example of perfect health and vitality. When I was almost 39 years old, I married a young woman who was almost 22. People told us that it would not work, due to our difference in age.

Despite this large difference (almost 17 years), I have never had the slightest difficulty in keeping up with the energy and vitality of my young wife, even after 25 years of marriage. The factors that are responsible for good health are many: liking life and liking myself, maintaining a balanced, healthy, and positive emotional psyche, correct and adequate nutrition, regular exercise, discipline, and an intense spiritual life.

According to specialists, most illness is of psychosomatic origin, and is also provoked by nourishment deficiencies caused by inadequate eating habits or aggression against the body.

I have accompanied much research and many studies concerning the health situation of the world. Rather than comment on the results of these studies, I decided to do my own research, so that I could personally verify the results. For this I separated people into three distinct groups: healthy, somewhat healthy, and sick. Their ages ranged from 15 to 50 years.

The results indicated that 65% of the group fell into the **somewhat healthy** category (and most of these were under 40). These people suffered frequent minor abnormalities such as tiredness of body or vision, head, back, and leg aches, poorly functioning digestive system, weakness, lack of appetite, breathlessness, dizziness, insomnia, frequent colds, allergies, and nervous problems.

The **sick** group came to approximately 4% of the group, and was made up of people who had difficult-to-cure diseases such as diabetes, cardiac problems, hypertension, osteoporosis, chronic rheumatism, etc. The remaining 31% were those who could be considered **healthy**, for they did not suffer any sickness or irregularity.

Those who keep up with world statistics about average life expectancies, have observed that the rates are falling in some parts of the world, even though recent research has indicated that the average life expectancy in many countries, of people over 70, has increased.

Studies in the area of medicine have shown that there has been an increase of the number of young people who suffer some type of malady, physical discomfort, constant illness, or some kind of sickness that hinders them from enjoying a healthy and pleasurable life. These problems have been attributed to lifestyle, environmental pollution, the deterioration of the quality of foods, and an agitated and undisciplined way of life.

I attribute this to the lack of self love and respect, lack of interest in caring for the body, indifference towards life, lack of information concerning how to preserve good health, an undisciplined and unruly life, incorrect and deficient eating habits, and the consumption of harmful products.

When I investigated the reasons for which certain countries have a large number of people who live to the highest age averages in the world, I discovered that this is due to the fact that these people carefully follow certain norms and natural methods of sickness prevention, and adopt the cares and formulas utilized by their ancestors.

Modern life and industrialization have been responsible for our abandoning many of the fundamental rules followed by our parents and previous generations, which helped people to prolong life and youthfulness. The cares and methods that I practice are practically the same as those who have reached high life expectancy levels.

When I turned 60 someone asked me, "How is your health today?" I answered, "Better than when I was between 20 and 25, because that is when I decided to adopt a correct life methodology, for I suffered from various irregularities and disturbances of my organs." In the past 15 years, though I suffered two serious accidents that resulted in spinal trauma, I do not know what it's like to even feel dizzy, nor do I remember the last time I had a cold, it was so long ago.

I owe this to an infinite number of factors, but the main one is the love and care that I have for my body, along with the great pleasure I derive from living this wonderful life that was given to me.

Nutrition: Fountain of Life, Health, and Energy

What we eat is the sustenance of life, health, and energy. If a person does not eat an adequate diet, in just a few weeks he will lose his energy, his health, and ultimately, his life. It is in the food that we eat that we find proteins, fats, carbohydrates, minerals, and vitamins. All of these nutrients are indispensable for the organism to be able to perform a series of functions that will determine the metabolic balance of the body.

The process of nutrition begins at the beginning of life, with the formation of the fetus. Nutrients in general are the main ingredients that allow the fetus to develop naturally, and which will determine the quality of health and a normal and healthy development. It is common for a pregnant woman to crave a larger amount of food. This happens because the being within her absorbs the nutrients from her organism.

Thus we can see that from the beginning of life, the human being needs adequate nourishment. The type of food adopted will play a vitally important role in determining a series of factors that will define physical structure, the structure of the organs, and mental health.

A lack of nutrients in the organism is one of the main causes of physical and mental deficiencies. Therefore, without an adequate diet, perfect and normal development is extremely difficult.

Nutrition is so important for the health and well being of the human race that governmental authorities are constantly on the alert to satisfy the needs of the population. Of all of the social problems that the world faces, food is the most urgent. Where there is hunger, it is impossible to solve social problems.

The discussion of nutrition is a somewhat uncomfortable one, considering that the majority of the world's population is unable to maintain an adequate diet. Besides the question of economic difficulties, many people do not know how to eat properly, are not interested in knowing about nutrition, or are unconcerned about following a proper and healthy diet.

As food is basic for a healthy life, and given the importance of the subject, currently there is varied and extensive literature available about nutrition.

Those who know a little about nutrition, know how difficult it is today to acquire healthful foods. Several factors have led food producers to utilize chemical additives.

Each day that passes it becomes more difficult to find vegetables or fruits that are free of chemical additives, which has led to the deterioration of the quality of food. Due to the poor quality of these products, and other factors concerning the problems involved in food conservation, even while following an adequate diet there is a health risk for the population. Even so, despite this fact, it has been proven that an adequate diet is the primary factor for good health, and, consequently, for living a better and longer life.

Most people, even those who enjoy a better social and cultural level, are unaware of what constitutes an adequate diet. I have read many books, taken courses, and listened to lectures about nutrition and aesthetics, and I have also gathered information from doctors and nutritionists.

Nutrition is an inexhaustible subject, and often controversial. Based on the opinion of specialists, and also on my own personal experience, adequate nutrition requires, in order to achieve balance of the metabolic system, the consumption foods from all types of nutritive substances: proteins, fats, carbohydrates, minerals, and vitamins.

When these nutrients are absorbed by the organism, each one has a synchronized and harmonious role to play so that the body can carry out its functions.

Here is an example. All human beings need a certain dosage of fats for the body, which are necessary for the formation of the cell membranes that transport vitamins A, D, E, and K, which provide the organism with the fatty acids that it is unable to produce for itself. Without these fats these vitamins would not be utilized (absorbed) by the organism, because they dissolve in fat. Therefore it is essential that we consume a regular amount of fats. The ideal is the dosage which corresponds to the daily necessities of each individual, for excessive fats result in imbalances.

Adequate nutrition consists of controlling the foods consumed, and taking the care, at each meal, to consume the quantities of nutrients considered ideal for each nutritive substance. It is also important to vary the types of foods frequently. It is very difficult to successfully obtain this balance. Despite all the knowledge I have acquired, it took me several years to find a diet that was ideal for meeting all of the needs of the organism, as well as conserve weight and healthful vitality.

Even so, sometimes I still find it difficult to get the balance right, especially when it comes to the quantity of carbohydrates, fats, and proteins. This would be much easier if I were not constantly concerned about weight maintenance.

Adequate nutrition does not mean just eating well and eating a variety of foods. It is also necessary that the foods consumed at each meal contain all of the ingredients that the body needs in order to fulfill its functions and to maintain perfect balance. It would be useless to eat well, yet consume only proteins, fats, and carbohydrates. The organism also needs minerals and vitamins in general. Otherwise, sooner or later, some imbalance will surface, causing disturbances and sickness.

It has been scientifically proven that adequate and healthy eating habits are responsible for many factors that determine the body's state of health, such as the formation a resistant skeleton and strong bones, good and strong teeth, strong nails, good quality blood, proper functioning of the organs, good and healthy skin, healthy hair, a good memory, good vision, resistance to sickness, and good health and vitality.

Energy Depends on Adequate Food and Physical Activity

Among the factors vitally important to the complex physical and organic constitution of the human body, in relation to health, is energy – the vital force that comes from within us.

The process of energy production is very complex, and involves a series of reactions of the organs. The energy produced by the body, which it stores, needs basic elements, which are the nutrients found in foods. These are the principal agents that generate energy for the body to store, and are also responsible for the vigor and vitality that determine physical strength and resistance.

When we study the process of energy production, we can see that the methods utilized for this physiological action can produce it in varying degrees, and according to the circumstances. It is influenced by the type of force exerted, its intensity and duration, and the individual's state of health and physical capacity, which is usually determined by the quality of nutrition, as well as other factors.

Those who study the mechanisms in the process of energy production have proven that people who practice regular physical exercise have a much higher capacity for energy production, for dynamic physical activity revitalizes the energy production system.

Physical exercise activates the circulation, facilitating the distribution of nutrients to the muscles and organs. Also, when the circulation is increased, the cells receive more oxygen, which, associated with other biochemical factors, contributes towards producing hormones and accelerating the metabolism.

The increase of the blood flow to the brain, resulting from physical exercise, brings about important benefits for cerebral activity. It helps to improve the mind and the psychological and mental state, as well as influence the process of physical energy production.

As the food consumed is the main factor for maintaining good energy, this has been the part of my method that has required constant attention. Assuring that daily nutrition is sufficient to fulfill all of the necessities of the organism is essential.

When I began this dietary control, and sought to eat a balanced diet, I encountered some difficulties concerning the dosage of the nutrients. It is a difficult thing to control, especially when one desires to control his weight. It requires in depth knowledge about nutrition. But over time, with daily practice, I was able to develop an eating program and a type of balanced diet that has allowed me not only to maintain the same weight, but also to enjoy this health, energy, and vitality that I consider to be excellent for someone over the age of 60.

In order to maintain good energy it is necessary to follow a healthy diet, practice regular and dynamic exercises, and maintain a healthy and balanced psychological and mental state. All of these factors work together towards good health and the preservation of youth.

Vitamins: Health and Balance For the Metabolism

A great number of people, regardless of their social or economic level, are unaware of the importance and necessity of vitamins for good health.

In the type of dietary regime I have followed for many years, what has demanded much attention has been determining the exact quantity of vitamins that should be taken daily. The human organism needs a relative quantity of diverse vitamins. Therefore it is necessary to alternate the types of vitamins, and to consume, at each meal, dosages that are sufficient for the necessities of the organism, depending upon one's activities for the day and his physical state.

In order to be able to arrive at this point, I needed to study extensively about nutrients. It is difficult for even an experienced specialist to determine whether or not an organism has a vitamin deficiency. This is possible through laboratory exams. With the knowledge I have acquired about nutrition, and day-to-day experience, I can now foresee the necessities of my organism with precision.

The best way to assure a vitamin supplementation that is closest to perfection is to follow a well balanced diet, seeking to consume foods that contain all types of nutrients.

I fully agree with the specialists and researchers who believe that a balanced diet, one that guarantees a perfect vitamin intake, will result in better health for the body. Correct vitamin intake makes it possible for the intestinal flora, and for the organism in general, to function properly, which provides good balance for the metabolism.

This is a very broad subject. New information is frequently becoming available about vitamins. With modern technology, new discoveries are being made about these nutrients that are so important for maintaining good health.

Studies have proven that the lack of these invisible substances, which we generically call vitamins, can result in a chain of diverse maladies: scurvy, rickets, sterility, cardiovascular disturbances, immunological deficiencies, anemia, weakness, and many others.

The most recent research has revealed that some types of vitamin deficiencies are responsible for mental imbalance and circulatory deficiencies, which causes the degeneration of tissues and contributes towards sicknesses that influence the aging process.

Many studies confirm that vitamin deficiency can produce a series of complications. According to these scientific studies, just the lack of a simple part of B complex, par-aminobenzoic acid, can provoke irritability, weakening of hair follicles, nervousness, headaches, depression, digestive disturbances, tiredness, and constipation.

Based on undernourishment experiments that I performed, using my own body, and on the examples cited, it is possible to have an idea of the trouble that can be caused in the organism by vitamin insufficiency, and the influence that they have on the process of health and energy maintenance, and on the control of metabolic balance.

By these examples we can also verify the great importance of a balanced diet, one that meets our vitamin needs. People who are accustomed to the traditional plate in our country (Brazil) – that is, rice, beans, and meat – will certainly lack the essential nutrients and vitamins necessary for maintaining a well-functioning organism and balanced metabolism, unless they supplement their diet with cereals, fruits, and vegetables.

When I feel that my body is in need of some specific vitamin, I usually take a natural vitamin supplement containing the vitamin in question, as well as other nutrients. I use either specific vitamins, or ones combined, for different situations, such as a preventative measure against colds or the flu, for recuperation from sicknesses such as throat or lung infections, for liver or intestinal problems, physical or mental stress, or loss of vitality.

According to studies made by specialists, a good and balanced, and carefully controlled vitamin supplementation, along with other nutrients, helps strengthen, recuperate, and reestablish the organism from various deficiencies, and also helps the regeneration, renewal, and prolonging of the life of the cells and tissues. This results in a healthy and resistant organism, which is essential for the maintenance of good health and for prolonging youthfulness and life.

An Adequate Diet

Before discussing what I understand to be an "adequate diet," I would like to make some clarifications. In order to follow any program, or nutritional diet, it is first necessary to undergo profound analysis and various examinations, accompanied by a nutrition expert, in order to check for any abnormalities that may exist. If a very slim person is unable to gain weight, despite an adequate diet, it is possible that he has some sort of abnormality. The same is true of an overweight person who eats little. In this case he may have a glandular or endocrine abnormality, or it could be the consequence of other factors.

An adequate diet is one that meets the requirements of the organism and, most importantly, acts as an agent of restoration of the deficiencies and abnormalities of the organs.

Nature is generous, and produces all that is necessary for health and for the survival of human beings. One of the things that amazes me is the fact that in nature's food we can find medicinal agents that are able to restore abnormalities and deficiencies in the organism. Many disturbances of the organs can be corrected by the consumption of specific foods and nutrients.

Based on my frequent experiments, I can guarantee that it is possible to cure liver or intestinal deficiencies, and even control many nervous and glandular disturbances. I suggest that those who desire more information read specific literature or seek a specialized nutritionist.

Many people have asked me how long I have followed this diet. Even in the beginning of my life, my eating habits were what I would define as adequate and healthy. I was born in a small town, and my family lived on a farm. We stayed there until I was 12, when we moved to another town, and, for another 2 years, lived in a place where we were able to maintain the same eating habits. We enjoyed the abundance of many nutrients: cereals such as oats, wheat, corn, beans, and soy; fruits and vegetables of all types; fresh milk, cheese, cream cheese, and butter; fresh eggs, meat, foul, and fish.

Sweets were made from natural fruit and sugar extracted from the farm, unrefined. Among the foods that were never lacking were sweet hominy and grains such as whole wheat and rice, fruit jellies, molasses, and honeys from various types of bees. In short, from even before I was born I received adequate nutrition, for it was customary for grandparents to orient their children as to how they should eat during pregnancy, so that their children would be born strong and healthy.

I remember that in my childhood, my mother would often fuss at me because at mealtime I wouldn't want to eat. She would say that I was very thin, and needed to eat, so that I wouldn't become sick. What she didn't know is that I always went to the garden and orchards, and would fill myself with fruits and vegetables. I always had a tremendous appetite for vegetables such as tomatoes, carrots, and sweet potatoes, as well as for raw ones like lettuce, watercress, chicory, and cabbage, seasoned with olive oil, lemon, salt, or soy sauce.

Fruits are my "weakness." If they were sufficient to provide all that we need, I wouldn't eat anything else. I have always eaten bananas, apples, papaya, avocados, pears, grapes, peaches, guavas, pineapple, plums, oranges, mangoes, figs, passion fruit, lemons, tangerines, etc. I drink fruit juice every day. According to my mother, even though I was one of the thinnest of her children, I had a surprising amount of energy and was very resistant to sickness. While my siblings would be in bed with colds, fever, sore throats, etc., I seemed to be immune.

I have lost count of the number of years that have passed since I last caught a cold. It is very unusual for me to have a cold, sore throat, or lung infection. At the first sign I begin to fight them off by natural methods.

Besides a healthy diet, there are other factors that contributed towards my having a healthy body and an organism that is resistant to sickness. The activities on the farm were intense, and began early – at 4:00 a.m. Right after milking the cows, we would take the milk to the cheese factory, and would occupy ourselves with the work in the fields, returning only after the sun went down. Almost all of our activities were in the fields and out of doors. This type of life, constantly exposed to the sun, clean air, to cold and to rain, usually barefooted and shirtless, was one of the factors that most helped to strengthen my organism.

My father taught his children, and expected their help in all of the tasks, from a very early age. Generally speaking, farm tasks require much physical strength and activity, which also contribute towards strong bones and general health, and resistance of the organs, especially when this type of activity occurs during the growth phase. All of my siblings who spent their early years on the farm, and followed a similar lifestyle, are healthier and more resistant than the younger ones, who were born and raised in the city, and who had other standards and habits.

The greatest proof that the type of diet, and the program that we have adopted in my home are correct, besides my personal experience, are the results obtained by my wife, our children, relatives, and other people I have counseled.

A Controlled Diet

Since diet is one of the most important factors for maintaining good health, it has been one of the parts of my method that requires special care. Discipline and constant attention to the quantity of each nutrient consumed during each meal are essential.

The quantities can vary depending on various factors and circumstances. This variation is based on the day's activities, the amount of physical and mental force exerted, the state of health, and the reactions and symptoms of the organism.

In order to follow a controlled diet, it is necessary to have ample knowledge of nutrition, physiology, and biochemistry, and to understand the process of the functioning of the body's metabolism, especially the function of the nutrients in general.

The basis of my diet consists primarily in controlling the quantity of proteins, fats, and calories in each meal. After that there is the control of carbohydrates, minerals, and vitamins. The balance of these quantities, according to correct standards, plays a tremendous influence on a series of factors in the organism, such as the balance of the metabolism, weight maintenance, and good health.

As a result of this nutrient and vitamin control, my weight increased just 3 kilos after age 25 (from 62 to 65 kilos). According to the World Health Organization, as well as generic tables used by specialists, at my age, and according to my height, I should weigh 5 kilos more than I do. I used age 25 as a basis, because studies have shown that it is between ages 25 and 27 that the constitution of the body is completed.

The motives that made me want to avoid gaining weight were the following: 1) a slim body usually means a younger looking one; 2) I believe that maintaining a proportional weight, under a certain limit, increases the chance of maintaining good health; and 3) with a slim body it is easier to conserve certain characteristics that many lose after the age of 40 – agility, speed, balance, muscular firmness, firm skin, etc. - all which contribute towards youthfulness.

The most recent scientific studies have proven that a slender body is less prone to circulatory sicknesses, and is more likely to maintain physical vigor and vitality. Besides this, people who are able to maintain weight proportional to their height are usually more elegant in appearance.

Weight control has many advantages, therefore it is worth any effort. I am one of 8 children. Besides myself, the one who gained the least weight after age 25 gained over 10 kilos. My wife, even after 25 years of marriage, 3 children, and passing age 47, has gained just 6 kilos, and has maintained the same physical appearance (physical type) of when she was 25.

When we were engaged, she had some problems stemming from anemia. After we were married she was healed, due to a change in diet. Besides following an adequate diet, she also added natural protein-based supplements, along with vitamins and minerals.

Among the many experiences I have had in the area of nutrition, besides my constant research, I worked for over 3 years with a doctor who was a specialist in aesthetics. During this time I had the opportunity to follow the treatment of various people with anemia, as well as those who had low resistance to colds, flu, throat infections, and other problems caused by vitamin and nutrient deficiencies. After adequate treatment with the prescription of an adequate diet and nutritionally balanced supplementation, the health of these people changed dramatically.

Based on day-to-day experience, I was able to adopt adequate nutritional control, which has enabled me to not only maintain my weight, but also to enjoy excellent health and vitality. Everyone in my family follows the same diet I follow, and we have always enjoyed perfect health and notable energy.

Up until the age of 50, I never needed to see a doctor. From 50 to 60 I went twice, for routine medical exams, which is advisable at this age. I needed medical care after a serious car accident, in which I damaged my spine, and one other time after a fall of nearly 3 meters. My youngest daughter, who is currently 19 years old, only received medical care during the first 8 months of life. The same is true of my other children. All of them enjoy perfect health.

In the past 35 years I have tried to rigorously follow the same nutritional habits. I have never neglected to follow certain rules, which I feel are fundamental. On certain occasions, such as at parties or a meal served outside of our home, when I have no choice of what is served, I try to eat as little as possible, or even not at all.

Anyone who wants to follow a healthy and balanced diet has to be willing to make sacrifices, know what to avoid, have self control, be interested, and have much willpower. When I began my dietary control, the first thing I did was list the things I considered to be harmful to my body. Some of the things I eliminated were hot and strong spices, coffee, refined sugar (I prefer sweeteners or brown sugar), soft drinks, artificial juices, alcoholic drinks, fried foods, and canned foods, or those conserved by chemical processes.

I adopted the habit of eating just the essential things, always being careful to eat enough, at each meal, to meet the daily needs of my body. Normally I control what I eat by means of meal plans, always using a wide variety of foods for each meal.

Before showing you the nutritional program I have adopted, I would like to emphasize that any nutritional control should be accompanied by a competent specialist, in order to avoid the possibility of future health problems. Despite all of the knowledge and experience I have acquired about nutrition, I follow nutritional guidelines set forth by the specialist and naturalistic doctor, Artenio Olivio Richter.

My Nutritional Program

In the attempt to follow a correct nutritional program, I eat three main meals a day, at predetermined and rigorously observed times. The first, and the most important, is between 6:00 and 7:00 a.m. The second is between 12:00 and 1:00, and the third between 6:00 and 7:00 p.m. After this meal I do not like to eat anything except water, juice, milk or soy milk, tea, or fruit. If there is a need for protein supplementation before bedtime, or if I get hungry, I eat a fruit, fruit salad, cereal with milk, or soy milk blended with fruits.

I have educated my organism to abstinence from 8:00 p.m. until the next morning. I usually do not get hungry between one meal and the next, since I use correct and balanced nutritional supplementation.

Just as the body needs rest in order to recompose itself, so does the organism. Therefore we need to give it a break. This long period of rest is necessary for the organism to be able to adjust itself, which is essential for the maintenance of metabolic balance.

It is much healthier to go to sleep lacking some nutrient than to lay down with a stomach full of food. That is why I consider breakfast to be the most important meal of the day, for after a fast the stomach is prepared to support a good, full, and complete meal. Thus the organism will be fueled to generate the energy necessary for the first round of activities of the day.

I will not describe in detail all of the menus that I follow, for that is not the objective of this book. But I will comment about the food and the main criteria I follow.

I begin the first meal with one or two types of fruit: papaya, banana, apple, avocado, etc. Next I have milk with some kind of cereal: oats, wheat germ, wheat bran, corn flakes, beer leaven with guarana powder, soy milk blended with fruits, or milk mixed with chocolate. In the morning I always have some kind of bread with butter and honey, or fruit jam, molasses, or some kind of glucose.

When I need a greater quantity of proteins and calories, such as on the days I exercise, I also add foods such as yogurt, cheese, peanuts, peanut butter crackers, oatmeal with guarana powder and brown sugar, hot corn or wheat cereal, and soy milk blended with fruits. These are the most common foods that I eat for breakfast, and I try to constantly vary the menu.

For lunch I follow the same criteria. I use two types of grain, whole grain rice with one of the following: pinto (or similar) beans, garbanzos, lentils, peas, or navy beans. I always have two vegetables and two legumes. I eat every type of vegetable and legume, except cucumbers. For protein I prefer chicken and fish, vegetable protein, soy meat, or an omelet with vegetables.

To complete the proteins and calories necessary for this meal, I usually eat some kind of dessert, such as cheese with honey or guava paste, sweet potato pudding made with milk and chocolate, cream cheese with milk sweet, fruit salad, oatmeal, hot corn or wheat cereal, avocado beaten with a little lemon juice, or bananas smashed with cinnamon, milk, and sweetener or brown sugar.

Between breakfast and lunch I rarely consume anything other than water or natural juices, unless I have the need of some vitamin or protein supplementation. If I do feel like eating something during this period, I eat fruit.

If I know that I will need to eat less for lunch or dinner, I will eat a plate full of salad, with vegetables and legumes, about 15 minutes before mealtime. Then I will eat normally. This is a trick to help moderate the appetite in order to avoid overeating.

For dinner I eat much less. Our favorite meal at home is legume soup with pasta or cereal. We always add a piece of meat, both for taste, as well as for increasing the amount of iron. After dinner I usually do not have dessert. After this last meal I only eat if I am going to participate in an activity that requires a lot of energy.

It is very important, especially for weight management, to practice self control at mealtimes. I usually eat about 80% of what I would like to eat. Many times I leave the table even though I feel like eating a little bit more. After a few minutes this desire fades and only returns when it is time to eat again.

I do not eat foods such as those available at fast food restaurants. I like pizza and pasta very much, but do not eat them more than 2 or 3 times a month.

Those who experience hunger between meals probably have some kind of nutrient deficiency, some disturbance in the organs, or a metabolic imbalance.

Mealtime, for me, is sacred. I never rush to eat, and am always one of the last to finish, for I rigorously follow certain rules. 1) I do not allow any thoughts that are incompatible with the moment, especially worries; 2) I sit in a proper position and relax. If necessary I do respiratory or head exercises; 3) I chew each mouthful completely; and 4) I enjoy to the utmost each food, even if it is a simple plate of beans, or bread with banana.

As I finish this chapter, I am somewhat apprehensive, for I remember the difficult times in my life, in which I even experienced hunger. I think of the people who may be reading this book who are unable, financially, to adhere to a healthy and nutritious diet.

I cannot conceive of a happy and healthy people, who desire a better world, when we are surrounded by innocent children and other human beings like ourselves, with the exact same rights and needs, but who are withering away in misery, and suffering terribly for lack of conditions to eat properly.

I would to God that the changes that are taking place in the world are a foreshadowing of a new era, one in which men will be overcome with love for their neighbors, and will cooperate not towards war, but towards providing food, peace, and happiness for all peoples.

The Consequences of Nervous Tension

Among the various factors that interfere with good health, there are some that do so indirectly. These are factors related to the psychic emotional state, which cause diverse reactions in the organism, and, in both the long and the short term, bring about serious consequences.

Nervous tension is among the factors most commonly indicated by specialists as being responsible for a series of negative events that are harmful to the body. It is also considered to be one of the greatest evils of the century, and one of the worst epidemics in large urban centers.

Affliction and nervousness generate nervous tension, which is revealed by diverse symptoms: agitation, undue moodiness, self exaltation, or irritability. Studies have shown that all of these reactions cause muscular tension, which reduces the blood flow, causes respiratory insufficiency, and other disturbances that interfere with the proper functioning of the circulatory and respiratory systems. As a result, the proper functioning of the other systems of the organism are hindered, causing sicknesses.

Many specialists have pointed to nervous tension as a leading cause of glandular and circulatory disturbances, arterial hypertension, heart failure, stroke, and other dysfunctions that lead to sicknesses such as gastritis, gastric ulcers, rheumatism, back and sciatic pain, insomnia, migraines, stress, exhaustion, and other, even more serious conditions. It is also considered to be one of the leading causes of the alarming increase of abuses of alcohol, tobacco, barbiturates, and other drugs that are harmful to human health.

Since I worked in the medical field for over 13 years, and my professional work was related to phyto-therapeutic treatments, I know that psychiatric hospitals are in more and more demand; clinics for the treatment of nervous disorders are always full, and people are seeking psychiatrists and psychologists with increased frequency.

If we were to verify the causes of the increased interest in this field, we would find that nervous tension is among them. The factors that unleash this emotional state are many: worry, fear, insecurity, noise, agitation, pressure, economic concerns, and neuro-vegetative disturbances.

There are many opinions about nervous tension, but the one that is most in line with my understanding is that of Professor Eliezer Pereira de Barros, philosopher, theologian, and specialist in psychiatry. According to him, nervous tension results from a state of extreme anxiety, which is a fruit of a materialistic society which seeks, voraciously and at all costs, the fulfillment of its desires in detriment to its spiritual fulfillment. Pride, envy, and selfishness are directly linked to the factors that cause fear and affliction, the principal causes of nervous tension.

There is a saying that goes like this: No one better to tell a story than the one who lived it. It is not easy to face financial difficulties, especially after the age of 50, and when one has already experienced reasonable financial stability. This is what happened to me.

Many people, especially those who live in large urban centers, find it difficult to live a balanced and stable emotional life. The times in which we live contribute greatly towards emotional crises.

Although I had faced many difficult periods and many deceptions, disappointments, and sadnesses, I always faced such situations without crisis, for I followed certain Biblical principles and rules for facing and overcoming emotional crisis, which always helped prevent my emotional psyche from being greatly shaken.

Psychological preparation is one of the items in my method. The first step in avoiding nervousness, irritability, agitation, and anxiety is to train the mind not to permit these negative factors to have a negative influence over your emotional state. The human being has the power to control his emotional reactions; all it takes is the desire to make the effort. Any person, over time, is able to be what he trains himself to be, if he conditions his mind to have self-control, or to be calm and patient, in order to be able to support, with serenity, day-to-day oppressions.

We have, in our minds, a very strong power with which we can revert negative thoughts into positive and healthy ones, and negative influences into positive ones. I say this based on personal experience.

After having experienced, many times, difficult situations, and having faced serious problems, which would normally shake the emotional psyche, I can say that I have good control, and have never needed to resort to escapes such as alcohol, illegal drugs, or even prescription ones, or to analysts or psychoanalysts. **I have never allowed negative things to negatively affect my emotional psyche, nor do I enter into despair... with God's help.**

It was precisely during these moments of tribulation and great anguish that I was able to relate better to myself, my wife, my children, and with other people. Many negative experiences through which I have passed have had their positive side, for they helped me to lose my pride and to overcome other defects in my personality. They taught me to give more value to spiritual things, and less to material things.

All of this has served to mature me, and to help improve my psychological balance, besides helping to develop my spiritual man. Experience has shown me that it is very difficult to face certain problems without spiritual support. I attribute this victory in my emotional life to many factors, the most important being the Word of God, which has been my basis of support, since age 25, for overcoming emotional crisis and calming storms.

Once I overheard a conversation between a doctor and a cardiologist, who said this; "On the bed in my office many famous people have lain – great, rich, and powerful men. When they are well, they are full of arrogance, pride, and valor. But when they are carried in after a heart-attack, half dead, weak, and pallid, they behave like frightened children. It's a rare one who does not cry out, 'Oh my God, help me!'"

Human beings are limited, and subject to psychological frailty. But because of arrogance and pride, he does not easily believe this. As long as he refuses to recognize his limitations, and seek external help in order to strengthen his spiritual dimension, it is very unlikely that he will achieve the emotional balance necessary in order to control his emotions and support the load of oppressions, without resorting to alcohol and other escapes, which, in the end, are harmful to the health.

My religious experience is what has most helped me to reach a balance in my emotional psyche. Besides praying and meditating on the Word of God, I try to avoid nervous tension through sports, exercise, social and recreational activities, art, philanthropic activities, an intense religious life, a harmonious home life with my wife and children, as well as a harmonious life at work. My greatest weapon against nervous tension is to train the spirit to be lord of my mind, thus making it possible to control the negative emotional reactions that can cause harm to the body.

I have observed, in my experience in public relations, that people who live in a constant state of nervous tension, who are always afflicted, agitated, nervous, and anguished, not only do not enjoy a healthy life, but also become unpleasant and ill-humored people, who age more quickly.

Worry, Anxiety and Depression: Poison for Health

Anxiety, another symptom related to the state of emotional psyche, arises as a consequence of psychological disturbance and negative influences. Anxiety produces anguish, usually accompanied by painful oppression. Anguish is a state of profound disquiet, which oppresses the heart, affects the mind, and often leads to depression.

One of the most common symptoms of people who suffer from anxiety and are always afflicted and anguished, is the constant sensation of smothering. The agony caused by this sensation, besides making people unpleasant, bitter, argumentative, and predisposed to emotional crisis, also causes negative reactions of the body and health.

Specialists in the causes of anxiety, anguish, and depression, point to fear, despair, and apathy as the primary causes. It is common in our day for people to live in fear – the fear of violence, robbery, unemployment, the future, sickness, death. Fear in general causes physical symptoms such as muscular tension, rapid heart beat, trembling, lack of air, back pains, insomnia, difficulty in concentration, and apathy. All of these things prevent a healthy and pleasurable life.

Studies made by the psychoanalyst, Eliezer Pereira de Barros, who has done research for over 60 years on the causes of oppressions that generate anxiety, show that its origin lies in negative thoughts that are repressed in the unconsciousness. According to Barros, it is very possible that the anguished person lived in a hostile environment in early childhood. Upon reaching adulthood, everything that was introduced into the unconsciousness influences his character, personality, and behavior. Barros believes that there are people who, due to hereditary and environmental factors, are victims of deeply etched thoughts that exercise dominion over certain areas of the personality, causing disappointments that lead to anguish, which is the beginning of depression.

Those who live in a constant state of anxiety, besides running the risk of being the victim of the maladies that come from anxiety, also are subject to committing acts that are not normal or appropriate for people who are psychologically healthy and balanced. "No one can escape himself, and most people do not possess, in themselves, the strength necessary to remove from the unconsciousness the negative thoughts that enslave and perturb the mind, without outside help," affirms Barros.

Since I had a very turbulent childhood, because of family environment and several problems that I encountered in my adolescence and youth, which led me to rebellion, frustration, and complexes, I had much difficulty in achieving psychological balance. I had to read self-help books about psychology, listen to lectures, and even participate in transactional therapy. But of all these things, what helped me the most in my search for perfect emotional balance was my religious experience.

I still remember what I heard a preacher say, many years ago: "The human being has a soul, which sometimes needs inner healing, and a spirit that needs nourishment. And this is possible only when we are in harmony with God. Healing of the soul usually requires special treatment and outside help. And spiritual nourishment is essential for the body to have the energy it needs to support the load of oppressions that this turbulent world throws upon us."

During the phase in which I faced an identity crisis, and experienced moments of affliction and despair, I sought spiritual nourishment, and it was there that I found the solution. In this search I tried several different religions, such as spiritualism and oriental cults, but none of these filled the void that I felt in my soul - until the day that I decided to believe the Word of God, and follow certain principals. Some of these are: *Do not be anxious for anything, but make your requests be made known to God, through prayer and supplication, with thanksgiving in your hearts. And the peace of God, which surpasses all under-standing, will keep your hearts and minds in Christ Jesus.*" (Philippians 4:6-7).

The Word of God shows us that man possesses a spirit, and that this spirit must be developed and trained in order to dominate the manifestations of the mind and the desires of the body. To develop the spirit means to prepare it to control the emotional and sentimental reactions. Through the Word of God we can see that the Creator established principles and standards for His creation. The origin of suffering and oppressions are usually related to the non-fulfillment of the principles established by the Creator of the universe Himself.

The Bible shows us that man's indifference towards God, and his conduct that deviates from the standards of God, are the main causes of inner disharmony and the lack of peace, which generate all of the inner conflicts and oppressions that perturb and enslave the human mind, making a healthy and happy life impossible.

The methods that I use to resist and fight against things that bring oppression are: 1) prayer and meditation on the Word of God; 2) the reading of books that inspire healthy thoughts; and 3) the reaching of personal goals, such as courses, healthy social encounters, social work, etc. I have participated in praise groups at church for many years, and have written songs and poems; I read edifying books and write; I practice leisure and sports activities; I enjoy constant communion with my wife, children, family, and friends; I am always careful to create a harmonious environment in my home and workplace; I always try to treat people with love and respect. Besides all this, I try to remain at peace with God, with myself, with life, with other people, and with the world, regardless of the circumstances that surround me.

There are those who would question religion; however, it is impossible to contest something that has such long-standing results. I have been following Biblical principles for over four decades to maintain psychological balance. Though I have experienced many difficult moments, and times of sadness and bitterness, and many moments of anxiety, anguish, indignation, and disillusionment, I have never fallen into depression, for I always ran to God, where I found shelter and consolation. I would like to share one of Jesus' promises: *"Come unto me all you who are tired and heavy-laden, and I will give you rest. Take on my yoke, and learn from me, for I am meek and humble of heart; and you will find rest for your souls. For my yoke is easy and my burden is light."* (Mat. 11:28-30).

This recipe has never failed me, nor has it failed many other people that I know. It's a shame that most people do not want to receive the treasures that God puts at our disposition, hidden in His Word. They seek refuge from their emotional crises in philosophies, cults, and religious mysticism, which not only bring no solution, but also hinder them from having a real experience with Jesus Christ, the only way that I found for a life of true peace, joy, and happiness.

I do not say this based solely upon my own personal experience, but also upon the experiences of millions of people throughout the world, who would say the same thing. Instead of seeking the right way to freedom from emotional crisis and depression, millions and millions of people remain victims because they prefer to give themselves over to pleasures and vices such as alcohol, stimulants, antidepressants, tobacco, sex, and other avenues of escape that naturally serve to aggravate the situation, and to generate yet greater anguish and suffering, which are hindrances to a happy and healthy life.

Ill Humor: Agent of Early Aging

Some of the qualities that most contribute towards beauty and a meaningful life are friendship, community life, the practice of fraternal love, respect for other people, and good humor. Anyone whose life does not reflect these concepts most likely has a disenchanted, meaningless, existence.

An ill-humored person is, by definition, not a friendly one, and can even be quite unpleasant. Therefore it is common for him to become solitary and isolate himself from others. This attitude is not healthy, and reveals maladjustment of the psychic order. Even though the personalities of these individuals may vary, their behavior is generally very similar.

There was a time in which a stern and serious face was a symbol of authority and manhood. But today we live in the greatest period of social and cultural explosion, when knowledge is breaking all barriers, especially in the areas of science and general know-ledge. Why then, so many ill-humored people? As I understand it, this mania of sullenness and ill humor are things of the past. It is a clear indication of mental under-development.

But unfortunately, when we investigate the causes that make a person become ill humored, we can find many justifications. We live in days that require a great struggle to achieve a space, a place in society, and a better position. Social and economic inequality have so oppressed the human race that it has influenced even his character and behavioral formation.

The day-to-day struggle against the difficulties and oppressions that affect us, besides affecting our psychic and emotional well-being, also dulls our affections, and even our interest in interpersonal and social relationships. The struggles and thorns that we face in life, coupled with pride, arrogance, presumption, and envy, have made many people insensitive and hardened, affecting their humor and corrupting spirituality.

A person's humor reflects what is inside him. Bad humor can be generated by personal dissatisfaction, nonconformity to the realities of life, hostility, traumas, and psychological symptoms such as hurt feelings and bitterness, deceptions, revolt, hatred, and resentment. Professor Eliezer Pereira de Barros says, in one of his lectures on psychic problems that every ill-humored person needs help, and that ill humor reflects the affliction, anguish, indignation, and sadness that are hidden in these people.

I know many people who, when they were young, were full of life, always happy and content, and good humored. But over the years they have become hardened, unpleasant, and ill humored. There are examples in my own family.

I made this observation to show how people can become ill humored. But my point is that ill humor contributes towards premature aging. There are many reasons for this. One is because ill humor dissipates some of the characteristics of youth; such at good humor and happiness, and the person often becomes unfriendly. When this happens, it is a sign that something is wrong internally; it's the manifestation of a psycho-physical illness, which results in a person's getting "older."

Over the years I have analyzed friends and relatives who are customarily ill humored, and have been able to affirm that all of them, including some under the age of 30, have disturbances that affect both physical and psychic health. Among these are gastrointestinal disturbances, constipation, gastritis, gastric ulcers, muscular tension, back pains, nervous and circulatory disturbances, and apathy.

It is interesting to note that most of these people were victims few undesirable situations, and had not suffered serious deceptions and disillusionment, compared to what I have suffered. I say this because normally it is frustration, disillusionment, and failure that bring about ill humor. Most of the people involved in my research were over 40, and had already achieved satisfactory social and economic positions. Even so, they were constantly given to ill humor.

Another reason that ill humor causes premature aging is that ill-humored people always scowl. Thus the facial muscles are constantly contracted, causing well-defined wrinkles to form even before the age of 40, and certainly by the age of 50 these people appear to be much older than they are.

The face is naturally the most visible part of the body, and also the most important when it comes to physical appearance. It is our face that people see when we introduce ourselves. It is the mirror of a person's interior.

The great wise man, Solomon, said, "A man's wisdom makes his face shine, and softens his features." In other words, scowling and ill humor are signs of a lack of wisdom; that is, being unwise.

If we train our inner man to be unfriendly, bitter, insensitive, and cold (unloving), this will reflect in our facial appearance, and will influence our manner of being. But, if we act with wisdom, and train our inner man to practice positive things such as love, kindness, politeness, sympathy, and cordiality, so that we can enjoy good interpersonal relationships and always be in good humor, we will be rewarded with a happy and jovial appearance. This is a positive step towards maintaining a healthy life.

Youth: Phase or State of the Individual Spirit?

Youth is one of the most interesting and beautiful phases of life. It is a period in which the body reaches the height of physical beauty, health, vitality, and energy.

The word "youth" can be defined as a state of joviality in which the manifestation of distinct characteristics, those pertaining to a youthful age, occur. Young people should be, by nature, happy, enthusiastic, cheerful, gracious, good humored, and communicative, for the joviality of a person is reflected by the manifestation of these characteristics. There is something wrong with a young person who does not display these characteristics. They are possibly the victim of psychic trauma, or have some other type of serious problem. To say that a young person who is always scowling, and does not like to show joy or good humor, does so because of his temperament, is unfounded. This type of young person is not normal or healthy, from a psychological standpoint.

To preserve youthfulness is to maintain the characteristics of this remarkable phase called youth, and especially to cultivate the natural attitudes of a normal young person.

We have the custom of determining an age range that we call youth, but there are no age limits to being jovial. It is not uncommon to find mature people who get along well with young people, and participate in any event with the same disposition, vitality, interest, enthusiasm, and dynamism.

In order to be jovial, one has to have a jovial mind. Healthy young people should naturally be excited, full of enthusiasm, uninhibited, spirited, and happy. Not everyone manifests all of these characteristics, for differing reasons. What most influence the state of spirit of a young person are the problems he faces day-to-day, and the negative experiences that mark his personality.

Many adults, despite their age, conserve the same jovial spirit they had in their youth, and show this in their way of behaving, thinking, speaking, and even dressing. Despite the years that have passed, their manner of being does not change.

On the other hand, many young people, upon reaching the mid-20's, begin losing the spirited and uninhibited ways that had been characteristic of them. It is common for their personalities to change once they begin adulthood and begin facing the difficulties that normally arise at this beginning of their independence. Thoughts about what they should be or achieve, uncertainties about the future, and anxiety related to obtaining financial independence, along with the difficulty of daily struggle, make many young people mature too quickly, and lose the peculiarities of their youth.

Many people, while still young, once they get married and assume greater roles of responsibility, become so serious that they quench the playful spirit and lose the graciousness they once had, along with their good humor and joy. Others become totally disinterested in their personal physical appearance. Some withdraw to such a degree that they lose interest even in recreational and social activities.

I have always loved making friends, and I know people like few people do. I have a very large circle of friendships. Among my closest friends, I have friends from various age groups. This makes it easy for me to make conversation that is interesting for the different groups. Among these people are friends who are near my age, between 58 and 63 – these are my friends from childhood. I met them when I lived in a small town, and we grew up together and have maintained regular contact.

At the age of 23 I moved to the city of Sao Paulo, where I made another large group of friends between the ages of 20 and 25, who are currently between the ages of 60 and 65. I enjoyed the friendship of these people between until I was 32, when I moved to a smaller city. Once again, very soon I had a new group of friends. With this new group an interesting thing happened. Even though I was nearing 33, people thought I was between 17 and 20. So I chose to spend my time with young people between the ages of 18 and 25 – people who are currently between the ages of 48 and 55.

Since I have always looked younger than my age, I have always had more contact with people younger than myself. Today my friendships range from ages 35 to 65. I attribute this to the jovial appearance that I still maintain, but most importantly, to the fact that I have never stopped manifesting youthful behavioral characteristics.

The fact that I look younger than my age has allowed me to spend much of my adult life among young people, which is something that brings me great pleasure. I have always gotten along well with younger people, and have experienced humorous situations. Once I went to watch a play that I did not know was prohibited for minors. The doorman would not let me in until I showed him my I.D. At the time I was 36 years old. Many were the times that I had to present my I.D. in order to prove my age, and prove that I was not lying.

Since I am already over 64, I have the right to preferential treatment for the elderly, guaranteed by law. Every time that I enter into this line in banks, or in other public organs, I am obliged to show my identity, and it is not unusual for others in the lines to get upset with me, because of my youthful appearance. I could relate innumerable stories of this type, but I will put aside references to physical appearance in order to emphasize the aspect related to the mental and spiritual.

One of the reasons that I enjoy being with younger friends, is that my older friends, especially those my age, with few exceptions, already act like old people. They don't participate in life's events with the same enthusiasm, interest, or disposition. It seems as if many people get old because they want to. These are the ones who destroy themselves physically, psychologically, and spiritually. I usually say that in life, everything depends upon self discipline and practice. If you train yourself to be playful, happy, and spirited, and take care of your body in order to maintain a youthful appearance, mind, and behavior, you will certainly be successful.

However, those who prefer to exert no effort, be ill humored, and live with a scowl on their faces, thus erasing the characteristics of youthfulness, will certainly be that which they want to be, and will appear to be old, even while young.

It is exactly this predisposition to preserve a jovial mind and spirit that maintains the will, disposition, and interest in taking care of physical appearance, and, as a consequence, this contributes towards conserving the characteristics of youthfulness, even after passing middle age, and entering into old age.

An Undisciplined Life Accelerates Aging

Since I have lived in several different cities, I have had the opportunity to meet hundreds of people, of different types, races, and customs. And as I have worked for many years in contact with people, always in the area of public relations, I have become an attentive observer, and am constantly analyzing people's behavior and attitudes. Therefore I can affirm that the majority live undisciplined lifestyles, while the number of people who do establish rules of discipline for their daily lives are a small minority.

In very few instances have I found someone who lives his life by correct norms, regardless of his social status. Whether or not one follows certain rules is a question of will, interest in life, and enlightenment. Those who make it a habit of practicing discipline, and following discipline with interest and dedication, are saving themselves from inconveniences that could be experienced by their bodies and health, and are healthier than those who follow no such disciplines.

One of the first things I did when I decided to follow a method was to adopt a series of disciplinary norms. To establish rules means to control the factors that significantly influence physical and psychic health, such as diet, rest, recreation, hygiene, and vices.

Diet is a key factor. I am one of those who believe that most sicknesses begin at the mouth, for it is through the mouth that foods enter that generate a multitude of disturbances, as well as sicknesses.

In an evaluation that I made, based on information about dietary habits in various countries, I was able to prove that the number of people who adopt methods for controlling the quantities of food, and the manner of eating, is very small. I could affirm that the majority of people, of all social classes, do not worry about controlling either the quantity or the quality of their food. There is very little information and interest in controlling these two factors. Many do not observe regular times, or intervals between meals, and eat too quickly, and in excess.

Undisciplined eating habits are the main cause of diverse disturbances of the organs, which cause many diseases, affecting the digestive, intestinal, glandular, and circulatory systems. One malady leads to another, until the body reaches the point of true calamity. And all of this simply because there is no concern about controlling the diet.

Another factor of vital importance that few observe, especially while young, is rest. I can still remember many of my peers who would spend night after night partying and drinking, while getting up early the next day to go to school or to work. They would do this for months on end. Many adults also follow the same course; they go months and even years without adequate rest.

While a person is still young, he does not feel the results of inadequate rest. However, when he reaches his 40's and 50's, the consequences begin to manifest themselves in diverse manners, according to studies made by geriatric specialists.

When we think of rest, we immediately think of sleep. To obtain adequate rest it is necessary to always observe the correct time for sleeping, and also to train the mind to eliminate thoughts and relax the body. The organism needs to reach the stage of deep sleep in order to be able to revitalize its energy.

I consider recreation to be a vitally important factor for health, for it serves as an escape valve. For a happy and pleasurable life, leisure is indispensable. Recreation is going for a walk, practicing sports, spending time with friends and family, and being involved in interesting hobbies that distract the mind and renew the emotional psychic state. In short, it is performing activities that release tension and bring satisfaction to the mind and spirit.

Many people take the easy way, and waste many precious hours, which should be dedicated to leisure, in front of the television, often filling their minds with negative and useless things. Or they spend their time reliving negative things that do not edify, things of the past that do nothing to nourish the spirit, and even cause disquiet – a lack of peace – which results in boredom, when they could be nourishing their minds and souls with good, positive, and healthy things.

When I speak of hygienic habits, I do not refer merely to the care that we need to take of our bodies, but also to the hygiene we need to practice in the environments where we live, and where we spend most of our time. All that can be done to improve hygiene will result in health for our bodies and our general well-being. The lack of hygiene is responsible for many sicknesses.

When I speak of vices, I refer to those that are harmful to the health, such as tobacco, alcohol, and toxic drugs. There are many who believe that tobacco and alcohol are not harmful to the health if consumed in small quantities, or only sporadically. There is a divergence of opinion among specialists, and so any discussion about this subject would be controversial.

As I consider this subject to be of fundamental importance for those who desire to live a healthy life and preserve youthfulness, and considering the great influence that these vices have over the lives of millions of people all over the world, I will discuss my opinion in the next chapter.

Avoidable Vices Damage the Body

Anyone who would like to investigate the factors responsible for the increase of diseases, especially those that affect large numbers of people all over the world, will certainly find that many originate from the vice of tobacco, alcoholic drinks, and toxic drugs that are harmful to health.

Of all of the studies and research I have read on tobacco use, I consider those done by the World Health Organization, which has been widely divulged by the media, to be outstanding, as well as the excellent work done by Dr. Edson Ferrarini, concerning toxins and alcoholism.

After all I have read about the vices associated with tobacco, alcohol, and toxins, and after having accompanied many cases, I can affirm, without a doubt that these vices are harmful to the health, and contribute towards the degeneration of the body, and speed up the aging process.

I have heard people say, "No one dies a minute before their time!" People who say that think that we have a set day to die. I do not agree! I believe that people who constantly poison themselves, and act aggressively against their bodies, are anticipating the day of their funeral.

Despite all of the information available on these subjects, many people do not understand the harm that these vices cause the organism. However, many drug users, even knowing of the harm caused by tobacco, alcohol, and illegal drugs, remain indifferent and continue smoking, drinking, injecting, or otherwise consuming drugs. This is a tremendous lack of respect for life, and of love of self and of the body, besides being a clear demonstration of senselessness and foolishness.

It has been said, "All problems of vices are related to psychological imbalance. This may be personal insecurity, need of self-affirmation, an inferiority complex, fear, anguish, or an escape from reality." I agree with this and believe that a person, a human being who is unable to free himself from a vice, besides lacking the equilibrium necessary for self control, is weak and worthy of pity.

I do not say this with the intention of causing indignation, but I say it in order to awaken those who have these vices to reflection. He who was born to be a champion should not be defeated by a simple piece of paper with tobacco in it, or for glasses full of liquid with alcohol in it, or for a half dozen chemicals (drugs) contained in a pill or an injection.

For me, a true man or woman is one who knows how to say a firm "NO" when it's time to make a decision, in order to avoid, either in the long or short term, destroying their life or their health. Those who plan on living to a mature age in good health, on prolonging their youthfulness, and on living their days free of distastefulness and suffering, should keep themselves from anything that would harm their bodies, especially these vices that I have mentioned.

The Holy Bible affirms that the unwise die early for lack of prudence. That which a man adopts and practices in his life conduct, will, over the years, establish whether his body will enjoy good health, or whether it will be constantly committed to illness. The well-being of the body in the future depends greatly on the type of care and treatment bestowed upon it in the present. He who desires a life without unnecessary stress, and desires to enjoy perfect health in maturity and old age, cannot forget the first principle: **love and care for your body.**

It is common to hear this type of comment: "My grandfather smoke and drank all his life, and was over 80 when he died!" I usually retort, "He lived into his 80's? Well, he should have lived into his 100's!" I seriously doubt that these people did not suffer as a consequence of these vices, unless they just happened to die by heart attack or such, before feeling the results of the vices. But vices kill people. I don't say this just for the sake of saying it. I base my statements on what medical statistics have shown.

I have accompanied dozens of cases of people who have smoked and drank for many years. Some time ago a neighbor of mine died, after having spent several months in the hospital. Both of his legs had to be amputated because of thrombosis caused by the toxins in cigarettes. This man was just 56 years old, but his body was practically decomposing because of this vice, and because of the wounds in his stomach and cirrhosis of the liver caused by the vice of alcohol.

The consequences and pain suffered by people who, at middle age or later in life, fall victim to pulmonary illnesses such as chronic bronchitis, emphysema, cancer, or brain damage, as a result of tobacco abuse, are terrible things. At the end of life, years of agony are much more painful and sad. The same is true of the victims of alcohol, who have digestive ulcers and cirrhosis.

As for illegal drug abuse, only those who are first-hand witnesses know how much an addict suffers. How many terrible consequences and how many lives prematurely taken because of drugs! I have heard people say things like, "I smoke, drink, and use drugs because they bring me pleasure!" What good is such momentary pleasure, when later on it will bring sadness, suffering, and pain for the body?

There is some divergence among specialists. Some thinks that the "less harmful" vices, such as smoking and drinking, in small doses, do not harm the organism. Others think that either of the two, regardless of the quantity, will, over time, eventually cause serious harm. And there are yet others who think that smoking and drinking only cause harm when done excessively and continually.

Personally I believe that our bodies naturally accept everything that is beneficial to them, but reject all that is harmful. As the body has an exceptional capacity of adaptation, it takes some time for it to react to the things that attack it, even when these things are as harmful as the toxins in tobacco, and the chemicals in alcohol and drugs. However, suddenly, as if screaming out in revolt, the body manifests itself through sicknesses that eventually lead to premature death.

Despite the extreme importance of the subject, given the fact that health and life are at risk, millions of users of these products are not in the least concerned, nor do they want to learn of the harm that is occurring. The reality is right there, before the very eyes of those who do not wish to see.

Of all the problems that health authorities need to solve, smoking, drinking, and drug abuse are the most important, for they have cost public funds tremendous amounts of money, and caused terrible damage in the lives of millions and millions of people all over the world, not to mention the frightening number of premature deaths caused by these vices.

Results of an Undisciplined Life

As part of my research, I customarily make observations and studies on dozens of people with whom I have personal relationships, including relatives and friends over the age of 35, for the purpose of evaluating their state of health and verifying the physical changes that have occurred over the years.

If man's biological age limit is 120 years, I conclude that any healthy person who habitually protects himself, and lives in a disciplined manner, should be able to reach the age of 80, 90, and even 100 in good health. Diverse studies in the areas of geriatrics and gerontologists have shown that this is possible, as long as certain cares are taken, along with certain norms of discipline, from an early age.

Most of the people I accompany as research subjects are people who I have known since childhood and adolescence. I spent my childhood, adolescence, and part of my youth in a small town. Since I always liked to have a very active social life, I met many people and made friends with whom I maintain contact to this day. When I was a teenager I was part of a group of friends made up of over 50 people. Many of these had known each other since childhood, or since grade school. I had these same friends during adolescence and during part of my youth.

As we grew, leaving adolescence and reaching a more mature age, our group began to disperse, and to form distinct subgroups, for at this point we sought to have closer relationships with those whose character and behavior were more like our own. The differences that led the group to sub-divide are ingrained into my memory.

The first group, and the largest, is what we would call the "rough" group. It earned this name because of the brawling, drinking, gluttony, smoking, and the participation in prostitution, which they considered to be the sum total of what life was all about. Among these were those who smoked pot and used other types of drugs.

The second group was a little more moderate, and numbered about 30% of the original group. Some of them smoked and drank, but in less excess than the first group. Most also enjoyed some degree of partying, and even visits to the brothel. At that time I worked at a well-established pharmacy in town, and it was not uncommon to sell medications to those in this group for venereal diseases.

The third group, and the smallest, was the one of which I was a part. Though we maintained friendship with the others, we preferred to keep more to ourselves, for we didn't smoke or drink – perhaps very occasionally at parties – nor did we like heavy partying. We had a different mentality and behavior. This group was made up of more moderate and sensible people, who preferred to follow certain principles, as well as to protect themselves.

Despite the differences of character and behavior, I never discriminated in my friendships, and maintained a good relationship with everyone. Even today I still have a large photo album of when I was a teenager, in which I appear with almost everyone from the original large group.

Thirty years later I went back to that city, where I had spent those teenage years, and I took with me those old photographs. I made a list of everyone in the pictures, with the objective of finding these old friends. I was able to find most of them, and the ones I couldn't find I was able to find out where they were and how they were through relatives and people who knew them.

One of the things that most called my attention was the number of these colleagues that had already died. In just one car accident 11 died at once. Two died in fights, three had died from drug abuse, and three more had died from either heart attacks or cancer. All of these who had died were part of the larger, "rough" group.

This proves that the things written in the Bible are true. The Word of God says that the foolish and irreverent will die before their time. All of these who had died had not been reverent with their parents, did not respect the law, and also practiced abuses in detriment to their health, which caused all sorts of troubles and inconveniences for those around them, such as car races, brawling, and other sorts of roughness.

As a result of this research, I also discovered the following: Of the "rough" group, I could not find one person who enjoyed perfect health. Some of them I had not seen for over 20 years, and were my age (50 at the time), but were unrecognizable due to the degree to which they had aged.

Of the second group, most were in fairly good health, though many had some sorts of sickness. The third group, of which I was a part, were all in very good health, with a better preserved appearance, and small health abnormalities.

In the "rough" group, the most common health problems, and symptoms of degeneration of health and of aging were the following (starting with the most common): vision deficiency, excess weight, circulatory and nervous disturbances, rheumatism, arthritis, arthrosis, back problems, baldness, lung disease, gastrointestinal disturbances (gastritis and gastric ulcers), hepatitis, prostate problems, impotency, stress, and loss of vitality.

Many people in the first and second group, who would sometimes make fun of us because we didn't want to participate in their antics, were amazed when they saw me, since I looked so young. The phrases that I most heard were "Man! You haven't changed a bit!" and "You don't get older!"

Among the people on my list for evaluation was a close relative, who is 5 years younger than me. He was part of a group that formed later on, but since he was tall, he would always hang around with older people. From the age of 14 he participated in the rough life, and enjoyed drinking and overeating. Today, when people see us together, they think that he is much older than I am. He looks older due to being overweight, white and thinning hair, wrinkles, the use of glasses, and even his posture. In short – he looks much older than his age.

The worst thing is not, however, his physical appearance. It's the serious physical problems he is already suffering, before reaching even middle age. He has a high degree of visual deficiency, arterial hypertension, back problems, rheumatism, arthritis, arthrosis, varicose veins, and high levels of blood sugar, cholesterol, uric acid, and triglycerides.

Why did this happen to this relative, and to so many others people that I know? Why do so many people have the appearance and bodies of people much older than their ages? Before responding I want to emphasize that I made this comment in order to alert future generations as to the importance of protecting themselves while they are young and still enjoy good health.

I can speak of this relative because we have been good friends since our youth, were constantly together until I was 25, and have always maintained contact. Even though we have a good relationship, our habits, customs, and lifestyles have always been very different. When I would go out with a friend or two or a girlfriend, he would go out with his group to parties and such. I would usually be in bed by midnight, or earlier when possible. He, on the other hand, would get home at all hours of the night, and almost always drunk. Sometimes he would do this for several days in a row. I remember, many times, seeing him come home at dawn, sleep for an hour or two, and then go to work. From work he would go to school. And it was common for him to leave school to go out with his friends again. His lifestyle always amazed me.

Other excesses also contributed towards the premature aging of this relative. Besides the drinking, he also smokes and has always eaten excessively and inadequately. He had gastric disturbances, but never worried about seeking treatment. Besides this, he didn't concern himself with adequate rest, was always nervous, became irritated easily, and had no interest in taking care of his spiritual needs.

Like him, many others told me that I didn't know how to enjoy life. But what are all these extravagances worth, if at just over the age of 50 one already has all of these health problems? Not to mention the possibility of dying at any moment because of hypertension, or some other serious health problem? Is possible that it was really worth it?

Obviously, not everyone would agree with me. What really was worth it was my determination to protect myself, and to live a moderate and balanced life, which has afforded me the privilege of passing middle age with a well preserved, jovial, and healthy body, as confirmed through the exams mentioned in the chapter "Analysis of the State of Health."

Ten Principles for Prolonging Youth and Life

After many years of study, research, and personal experience, I can guarantee that these ten principles that I have followed (in order of importance), are fundamental and should be adopted as basic rules by anyone who desires to maintain good health, and prolong life and youthfulness. They are as follows:

- Put God in first place, and fear and love Him above all things; obey all His commandments carefully, and live life of justice and righteousness.

- Give the greatest value to life, and always be grateful to God for the precious gift of life.

- Cultivate the gift of faith and hope. Always think and dream of good and healthy things.

- Like yourself, respect and take care of your body, and be humble in heart.

- Eat in a healthy and correct manner.

- Live a balanced and disciplined life.

- Regularly practice activities that exercise the mind and body.

- Develop a positive mentality; eliminate all that is negative, and exercise dominion over your feelings and emotional reactions.

- Always maintain good humor and joy, regardless of the circumstances.

- Live in perfect harmony with all relatives and other people, and always practice the following in your interpersonal relationships:

A. Love and friendship

B. Goodness and kindness

C. Affection and comprehension

D. Dedication and dialog.

The results that a person obtains in life are a consequence of his personal choices. Following these principles and basic rules is a matter of choice, of conscience, and of personal effort. Any person has the capacity to follow them; one just needs to put them in practice. The great American statesman, Abraham Lincoln, once said,

"It is no help to do for someone what he can do for himself."

I am not sharing these principles and rules because I think they might influence or help other people. I am sharing them because I am absolutely certain, based on my own personal life experience, and on the studies and research that I have been doing for many years, that if these principles are not followed, it is practically impossible for a human being to find the way to a full, happy, and healthy life, or to prolong youth and existence in this physical plane.

Conditions for a Peaceful, Healthy, and Long Life

After studying and observing the habits and behavior of human beings for many years, and analyzing their feelings and emotional reactions, I have no doubt that our bodies are made up of two other distinct elements: the soul and the spirit. The soul is the mind, the intellect. It is the fantastic and mysterious cerebral complex, the center of the emotions and feelings.

The spirit is the divine nature within us, but it is only perceptible to those who are spiritually sensitive, to those who believe and seek ways to develop it.

In order to have a healthy life, and one that is prolonged here on the earth, it is necessary to establish norms for taking care of the body, so that perfect psychological balance may be attained, and that the mind can be controlled, and the feelings and emotional reactions can be dominated.

Besides this, it is also necessary to develop the spirit, for the spirit should be the voice of command for the mind and body. I, my spirit, should say to the mind, "Be quiet, because the body is going to do what I determine." I cannot let my body do everything it wants to do. This liberality is exactly what has led so many people to a situation of physical and mental calamity.

When I became convinced that I needed to develop my spirit, I went to books and to many different sects, philosophies, and religions. Of all the formulas I studied, the only one that provided a coherent answer, and one that explained man's behavior, was the Holy Bible. Despite much meditation on other philosophies, I could find no answers to my questions and indignations. But the Bible, though so despised and questioned, gave me all the answers – yes, literally all of them.

It is a book that is full of revelations and instructions that will take a person out of the mediocre dimension in which he lives into another, much superior sphere, beyond that which is imaginable. The Word of God shows the way to live a fantastic and excellent life, full of incredible adventures.

Based on my personal experience, I can affirm that man is able reach such an elevated dimension in the spiritual realm that he is able to dominate his sentimental and emotional reactions, as well as sicknesses, and is also able to create a kind of "armor" against maladies.

The Holy Bible calls this dimension the "fullness of the Spirit" and "the fullness of God" (Ephesians 3:18-19) and "the stature of a perfect man" (Ephesians 4:13). This explains why Jesus Christ offered the other cheek when He was struck; because despite the fact that He was humiliated, tortured, and nailed to a cross by man, He was able to say, "Father, forgive them, for they know not what they do!"

This is incomprehensible to the human mind, but not to those who have reached this elevated dimension. This person understands that it is possible for a son, who loved his parents dearly, to receive the news of their deaths, and to dominate any emotional or sentimental reaction. Or to lose a brother, yet young (age 24), and not even cry. Or to learn that he has an irreversible disease, one that could put him in a wheelchair, and not be shaken. Or suffer six robbery attempts – four of them with threats of death – and in the end not lose anything material, much less his life. I say that this is possible because all of this happened to me.

The secret is in depth knowledge of the Holy Bible. But in order to reach this elevated spiritual dimension, there is a process established by God, and there are principles established by the Creator that have to be followed.

There are no drugs or drinks, nothing in this world that can bring the sensations and emotions that we feel when we seek in God a deep spiritual experience and an intimate relationship with Him. This is the only formula for filling the void that gnaws at the soul, and for bringing the inner peace that we all desire.

My opinion is not based merely on personal experience, but also on nearly 40 years of observation of many people who believe in the Holy Bible. There are millions spread out all over the world, who have discovered, in it, new lives – lives truly abundant, resulting in peace, joy, health, and happiness.

In the Word of God we find some conditions for enjoying a healthy and prolonged life. We can find examples in the book of Proverbs, which was written by the great wise man, Solomon, whom I consider to be a guide to peace, joy, and happiness – and consequently, to prolonged life. This we can see in the following texts from the Word of God:

Proverbs 3:1-2 - "My son, do not forget my teaching, but let your heart keep my commandments; for length of days and years of life and peace they will add to you."

Proverbs 4:10 - "Hear, my son, and accept my sayings, and the years of your life will be many."

Proverbs 9:11 - "For by me your days will be multiplied, and years of life will be added to you."

Proverbs 10:27 - "The fear of the Lord prolongs life, but the years of the wicked will be shortened."

Proverbs 11:19 - "He who is steadfast in righteousness will attain to life, and he who pursues evil will bring about his own death."

Proverbs 14:27 - "The fear of the Lord is a fountain of life, that one may avoid the snares of death."

Proverbs 15:10 – Grievous punishment is for him who forsakes the way; he who hates reproof will die."

Ephesians 6:2-3 - " ' Honor your father and mother' (which is the first commandment with promise) ' so that it may be well with you, and that you may live long on the earth.' "

In these few citations we can see a series of conditions established by God, followed by promises, for man to have a life of peace, health, and happiness, and for his days to be prolonged on the earth. Besides these verses there are many others that clearly show the great physical, mental, and spiritual troubles that come upon man, enslaving and destroying him, depending on his lifestyle. As a consequence of incorrect and unwise attitudes, problems arise that cause unhappiness and sickness, which lead to premature death.

The lifespan of each individual is not predetermined, but can be determined by his own actions. I have studied this subject in depth, and I fully agree that He who made us also had the right to destroy us whenever He so desires, or thinks it necessary because of our irreverence. I know that this is a difficult issue for many.

If a person's lifespan is determined by his attitudes, then why do so many die while still children, and innocent? The Bible shows us that God is sovereign over all things, and that there is a purpose to all things under heaven.

Peace, health, and a prolonged life depend upon norms that we establish for taking care of our bodies, and the criteria that we follow for controlling the mind and developing the spirit. But most importantly, it depends upon how we behave before men and before the Creator.

Man can attain the highest level of knowledge and intelligence, but if he does not believe that he has a spirit, and therefore does not seek to develop it, he will never have the wisdom and discernment necessary to discover his divine attributes.

The Bible tells us that the fear of the Lord is the beginning of wisdom. Those who do not fear or believe in God can never understand the spiritual secrets that give meaning to man's existence in this physical world.

If the Word of God affirms that the fear of God is the beginning of wisdom, it is also saying that those who do not fear God, and who ignore Him, will never have the wisdom that comes from above (divine wisdom), in order to be able to live their lives with intelligence and balance, to live a full and happy life.

The further away from God a person is, the less capable he is of controlling his emotional reactions. His animal reactions can manifest themselves mightily and in any situation, for his attitudes will always be subject to the impulses of instinct.

This type of person usually presents a low level of development and a high level of ignorance. Those who have a relatively high level of spiritual development because they fear God, have a much lower degree of animalistic reactions. And those who achieve an elevated level of spiritual development and conduct themselves according to the teachings of God, very rarely manifest animal reactions, regardless of the circumstances. This is because spiritual development results in self control.

These people have a high degree of wisdom and self control. Divine attributes predominate their minds, which influence all their thoughts and attitudes, resulting in a life of peace, health, and happiness, which are indispensable factors for prolonging life and youthfulness.

A Harmonious, Healthy, and Happy Life

First of all I want to say that the comments that I will be making here are not based solely upon my personal experience, but are also founded on the studies and research that I have been doing for many years. There are many factors that influence our state of spirit, and are necessary for us to be able to live a pleasure-filled and happy life.

One of these factors is peace, which is the most important one for inner harmony. The harmony that we enjoy will depend upon both emotional and corporal health. A harmonious and healthy life will result in a happy life, while a life without harmony or health is one without flavor or meaning, and full of tribulation.

It is often said that "Man lives in conflict," or "The human race lives in conflict." It is common in our day for us to label everything, and the conflict of man is no exception. There are many labels, but the most used ones are "existential crisis" and "identity crisis."

These so-called existential crisis, according to philosophers, psychoanalysts, and sociologists, has been the main cause of the increase in alcoholism, drug addiction, mental instability, violence, and suicide. This crisis does not chose the age or sex of its victims; they can be teenagers, adults, or even elderly.

Like many other normal people, I also experienced an existential crisis, and it was not easy. The causes of internal conflict are many. They can originate in the womb, or even more often, in childhood, in the home. Identity crisis, in general, arises from frustrations and day-to-day events that cause fear, hate, indignation, emotional wounds, frustration, disillusionment, emptiness, etc., which lead to states of personal dissatisfaction and depression.

Since we live in a day in which materialism rules, unfortunately man's worth is determined by his appearance, social position, or by what he owns. The attractions to material things dominate his mind to the extent that spiritual values decrease day by day, bringing forth this anguish that the human race experiences today. Crisis is mentioned in every sector of society.

The great crisis, however, is within the human heart. It is the inner conflict that generates disharmony in the family, and in personal and social relationships, that often provokes discord, war, disorder, and the unrest that reign in the hearts of men. Those who live in conflict with themselves and with the world usually do not accept life and are always predisposed to attract negative and undesirable circumstances to themselves.

For a period of several years I was the victim of inner conflict and problems of a psychological nature. These problems became more serious from age 19 to 25. I found refuge in alcohol, became depressive, and even considered the possibility of ending my own life. It was at this time that I realized that I needed external help. Thus began my search for answers through philosophies, sects, and religions, in the hope that I would be able to resolve my inner conflicts. Of all the types of spiritual help that I experimented, the one that helped me to encounter harmony, balance, health, and happiness was the Word of God, the Holy Bible.

Based on my personal experience, I can affirm that the first step to having a harmonious, healthy, and happy life is to be in harmony with the Creator (God). The second is to be in harmony with one's self. The third is to be in harmony with one's family and relatives. The fourth is to be in harmony with others. The fifth is to be in harmony with the world.

Some people have commented that I must have reached the age that I have with a youthful appearance because I have led a peaceful life, with no problems. To show that this is not the case, I am going to share some of the unpleasant chapters of my life, and, at the same time, show what it was that helped me to overcome my inner conflicts, frustrations, complexes, and the existential crisis that I faced.

Like many young people, I had problems in my family, and experienced some very difficult situations. I left home at the age of 16, no longer able to support the environment that existed there. Inexperienced, and full of revolt, complexes, and frustrations, I had a very difficult time adapting in jobs and with people. I reached the point of experiencing hunger and sleeping on the streets.

This went on until I was 23, when a relative, who was a businessman, decided to help me by giving me a job in his business in the city of Sao Paulo. As I was related to the boss, I was warmly accepted. This helped to minimize the frustrations and complexes I had as a result of the negative situations I had faced.

I had a very strong desire to succeed and to achieve a position in society. In less than two years I progressed up the social ladder, and acquired an excellent salary, a luxuriously decorated apartment, and a new car. This was a new phase in my life, and everything was going very well. I made many friends, went to good clubs and classy restaurants, bought whatever I wanted, traveled to many places, had nice clothes, and girls and parties were never lacking.

I was finally living all of the dreams that I had had as an adolescent. But despite the success, and the possession of all the things that I had desired, I felt a tremendous inner void. Nothing could satisfy me – not the friends, the girlfriends, the parties, the trips, or any other sort of pleasure.

The situation worsened daily. My unrest led me to seek more and more satisfaction in the pleasures of the world – the parties, the orgies, the drinks, the cigarettes, the car races – all of these only served to increase my depression.

It was at this point, when I was 25, that someone I had met earlier came unexpectedly to my home, and said, "You can have all the things in the world, and live all the pleasures that this life offers, but none of this will fill the void inside you. But there is someone who can, and His name is Jesus Christ!" I didn't pay much attention to what she said, for I had been searching for answers for months through Spiritualism and oriental philosophies, none of which had solved my problem.

I often thought of dying, and even contemplated suicide. Many nights I would spend hours driving around the city of Sao Paulo at high speeds, as if I were crazy, and often drunk, trying to commit "indirect" suicide, until one day I did suffer a violent accident. Though I was unhurt, I began to reflect about my life, and what was happening to me. That same night, lying on my bed, and unable to sleep, I remembered the words of that person had spoken to me, that only Jesus Christ could fill the void inside me.

The difficulties of my life had made me very rational and insensitive. For me to be able to believe something, I had to see it. But in the face of all that was happening, and because I had been unable to find a solution, on that sleepless night I decided to challenge God. I said, "Jesus, if you are real, are alive, and can help me to solve my problem, I am here, and I want you to show me!" Having said this I dozed off, and suddenly, as if I were dreaming, I heard a sweet and quiet voice say, "I am the way, the truth, and the life. No one comes to the Father but by me. Place yourself in God's hands and He will care for you."

I began to wake up. Since I had slept under the influence of alcohol, I thought that I had just dreamed, or hallucinated. But then I heard the voice again: "Your life is going to change. God has a great plan for your life; give your path to Him, and He will do the rest." I was unable to understand if what had happened was real or a dream. But I knew that something was happening. I began to feel something indescribable inside of me.

I opened the door to my veranda, which was on the 9th floor – the same veranda from which I had considered throwing myself some hours earlier. I looked up to the sky and began contemplating the moon and the stars. Until that day I had not liked the darkness of night, but at that moment I realized that the sky was beautiful and fantastic.

I began to feel a strong emotion, as if fire were invading my inner self. I felt, at that moment, the greatness of the Almighty, and the clear and incontestable sensation of the presence of the Creator. I fell on my knees and humbled myself before God, and began to cry profusely. I acknowledged that I was a sinner, confessing my sins, and asking God to forgive me. I said, "Jesus Christ, if you exist and are real, I ask you to fill this void in my soul."

I stayed there for a long time, laughing and crying at the same time, for I was feeling peace, joy, and happiness, such as I had never felt in my entire life. I remember as if it were yesterday, that extraordinary and wonderful encounter with God, and ever since that unforgettable day such experiences have been a constant in my life.

After this supernatural experience my life began to change radically. I stopped drinking and smoking effortlessly. I totally changed my way of being, acting, and living. My inner man was totally transformed, for whoever has a true experience with God naturally begins to manifest His character, and his conduct begins to reflect that of the Creator. The emptiness and void that I had felt in my soul, in my inner self, disappeared, never to return.

So that I would never doubt whether or not the experience was real, there was some clear evidence. For example, I had never read the Bible. At that time I did not know that the words I heard through that voice were to be found in the Bible: "I am the way, the truth, and the life; no one comes to the Father but by me," which is found in John 14:5. And "Place yourself in God's hands, and He will care for you" is found in Psalm 37:5.

Another piece of evidence is that after almost 40 years of living in fellowship with God, and after so many other, even more striking, intimate experiences with the Creator, I have no doubt whatsoever that it was not mere sleepiness or imagination, but a very real and true experience.

The greatest proof is the third piece of evidence: it is that I am here, fulfilling God's plan, and what was told me by that supernatural voice on that unforgettable night. I could never have imagined, at the time that after so many years I would be used by God as an instrument to share with others the message that one day rescued me from the path of destruction and death.

If I had not had a personal encounter with God, I certainly would not have arrived at this age with a healthy body or with the jovial appearance that I have, and I certainly would be suffering from many sicknesses. Or perhaps I would be dead, due to the lifestyle I led, or perhaps I would have committed suicide, as do so many who face the types of problems that I have faced.

The experience that I had with Jesus Christ, besides filling the void in my soul, also restored my physical well-being, and ended my inner perturbations, thus resulting in perfect emotional and psychic balance. It also freed me from vices, from complexes and frustrations, brought me inner peace, renewed my health, energy and vitality, and never again allowed me to feel solitude or fall into depression.

This materialistic world has made man a slave to pleasures that satisfy just the body. In this search for pleasure, man distances himself from God and from spiritual values, as he becomes more materialistic and lost in corporal pleasures. He forgets to seek that which would complete his spiritual self, and would fulfill the void in his soul.

This is what I learned after so many years of seeking something that would satisfy my spiritual man. The pleasures that the world offers for the satisfaction of the body and of the ego are temporary illusions, and end up bringing burdens. The search for pleasures that satisfy the body and soul (feelings and emotions), have led man to inner disharmony, despair, dissatisfaction, anxiety, stress, depression, mental illness, violence, and premature death.

Even after my personal experience with Christ I experienced many difficult situations, moments of suffering and sadness. I have suffered huge deceptions, been betrayed by people of my utmost confidence, been slandered, unjustly treated, humiliated, things that all people are subject to. But thanks to the inner force I found in God, I was able to face all of these difficult trials and "come out ahead," as the saying goes. Today I consider myself a WINNER, a happy person, and one who has achieved many of his dreams.

I have faced many difficult situations along the path of life, and many tribulations (even after the age of 60); after acquiring a large financial debt as a result of investment in an unsuccessful project; after receiving the news that I have suffered irreversible spinal damage, as a result of two accidents, that can paralyze both legs and leave me in a wheelchair. But in every situation I have been able to overcome the difficulties, seeking strength and help in God, and also because I have, in my mind, the most important quality of a winner – the determination to never be shaken or to quit, no matter how bad the tribulations and difficulties may get along this path we call life.

I believe that if it had not been for a strong spiritual structure, which has given me emotional balance to support all these trials, I would quite possibly be disillusioned with life, frustrated, oppressed, and disenchanted, as is the case with many elderly people. Also, this book would not have become a reality.

It was during moments of great weakness that I found strength in God to keep fighting. That is why I have been more than a conqueror, leaning on the teachings of Jesus Christ. All of the experiences that I have lived have served to show me that man is only exalted, made great, becomes wise, and has strength to overcome trials, barriers, the difficulties of life, and his internal conflicts when he discovers his divine attributes and begins to live life in trust and dependence upon the Creator, according to His teachings and principles.

There is a Bible passage that calls my attention: "What is man that you are mindful of him, and the son of man that You visit him? For you have made him a little lower than the angels, and you have crowned him with glory and honor. You have made him to have dominion over the works of your hands; you have put all things under his feet" (Psalm 8:4-6). These verses show the great value, the importance, that God attributes to the work made by His hands – the divine and precious creation called "man." But this divine creation, that can be crowned with glory and honor and taken to a superior level, has become prideful, and has neglected the principles established by his Creator. For this reason many people live mediocre lives that fall short of God's glory.

Man himself makes his own choices, for since creation God has given him free will – the absolute right of choice. To this day many people are far from God's glory, living miserable and insignificant lives, simply because, due to their self-sufficiency, pride, arrogance, and selfishness, they neglect God and His principles.

Millions of people spend their whole lives as "human rags," living in mediocrity, and without realizing that they have the right to a crown of glory and honor, and could be elevated to a position a little lower than God through reconciliation to Him through Jesus Christ. They go through life with their backs turned to God, living in disharmony with their Creator, because they lack the humility to acknowledge that without God's grace, they are nothing. They live and die without knowing of or enjoying what could truly be considered a harmonious, healthy, and happy life.

Is It Possible to Live a Serene and Pleasant Old Age?

Old age is a phase of life that many will have to face, like it or not. I am no different from anyone else, and so I, too, will one day live this phase. Despite all my care, and the fact that I have been able to maintain perfect health and a youthful appearance, some signs have begun to announce the arrival of old age.

Regardless of how much care is taken, as the years pass, slowly but surely signs of age will appear on the face, and changes in the body will become obvious. So, even with care taken to postpone old age, inevitably, sooner or later, it will come.

Once I was talking to a psychologist, and she told me that I should spend more time with people closer to my age, because otherwise I might find it difficult to accept the aging process. She said this because, as I have already mentioned, I like spending time with younger people. She told me that all of us have a natural psychological evolution, which happens gradually. I prefer being with younger people in order to retard this process of development, and to avoid problems in the future that would make acceptance of old age more difficult. So I answered, in a playful tone, "I know that! But I also know that the day that I think I'm getting old will be the day that I'm acting old!"

I seek to live intensely, without worrying about tomorrow. The Bible says, "Do not be anxious about tomorrow; sufficient is the evil for today." In other words, we have to be prepared to face today's challenges. I am not in the least concerned about old age, and I am sure that I will face that phase with serenity.

Even with all the care I take to prolong youth, I see old age as a natural consequence of life. A person like myself, who has attained a certain degree of maturity and emotional balance, will have no difficulty in accepting any of life's circumstances. On the other hand, the spiritual experience I have has led me to understand that many of the things so greatly valued in the world are merely illusion and vanity, and all are temporal.

I use my own life experience as an example. After so many years of study, research, and taking such good care of myself in order to prolong youthfulness and life, suddenly, when I received the sad news of irreversible spinal trauma, it seemed as if it were all for nothing.

However, this news did not shake me. I continue in peace and happy because I am prepared, both emotionally and spiritually, to naturally accept anything that might happen. This is because something exists that surpasses anything I might experience in this life; it is the hope of something much better, of a superior dimension, which surpasses any of life's experiences. It is the certainty of a new heaven and a new earth, promised by God to those who have received Jesus Christ as Lord and Savior (Rev. 21:1-4).

Many things that used to bring me pleasure, that I considered to be important, today I consider superficial. What makes many people, upon reaching old age, frustrated, disappointed, and disillusioned, is the simple fact that they did not achieve many of the things that they had sought in order to satisfy their personal and material desires. Without the hope of receiving something better at the end of life, old age will certainly be monotonous, sad, and burdensome. I can affirm this from the innumerable elderly people with whom I have had contact.

If I did not have this hope, based on God's promises, perhaps I, too, would have already begun to feel this burden. Up until this present date, even with all that I have achieved, the things of this life do not satisfy me, though I do feel a certain satisfaction in the fact that I have a successful marriage, four children, two daughter-in-laws, a son-in-law, and three wonderful grandchildren – all fruit of what I have sown.

After I came to the understanding that human happiness depends not upon material things, but upon spiritual, I learned to live better and happier, and life began having real meaning, despite the burdensome news that I received. And second to the spiritual factor, the most important factor for experiencing a pleasant and peaceful old age is the physical one. The person who protects himself and takes care of his body has three times the chance of other people to reach old age in good health. Otherwise this phase can be bitter and full of difficulties.

The Bible teaches that the burden and sadness that many feel in old age are reflections of acts practiced throughout life. It also shows that a man who behaves justly and righteously, who lives coherently and wisely, respecting other people and the laws of God, will naturally have a serene old age.

Biblical promises are always accompanied by a condition that must be fulfilled; you do this to receive that, you do that to receive this. It is the law of the Creator. First you have to do in order to then receive. Many people, even without realizing it, spend their entire lives practicing injustice, lying, cheating, deceiving, and committing dishonest acts that harm other people. They break the laws of the Creator with no concern whatsoever that one day they will have to give an account for their acts.

And there are also perverse people, who practice these things constantly. As for these, the Word of God guarantees that their old age will be accompanied by sadness, suffering, and burdens. This is only fair and logical! For each one will reap the fruits of that which he planted.

In the book of Ecclesiastes we find the following: *"Be happy, young man while you are young, and let your heart give you joy in the days of your youth. Follow the ways of your heart and whatever your eyes see, but know that for all these things God will bring you to judgment. So then, banish anxiety from your heart and cast off the troubles of your body, for youth and vigor are meaningless...Remember your Creator in the days of your youth, before the days of trouble come and the years approach when you will say: "I find no pleasure in them"* (Ecclesiastes 11:9-10; 12:1).

This passage shows some principles and conditions established by the Creator Himself, so that man can have a pleasant and peaceful old age. All of the serenity I enjoy, and the inner peace that I experience daily is the fruit of a profound and intimate spiritual experience with God. Each day I seek to have a more intense fellowship with God, and to faithfully follow the teachings of His Word, which reveals the only way in which a man can be lifted up to a superior dimension, and allow him to reach the end of his days fulfilled, peaceful, happy, and with the assurance of eternal life.

Personal Judgment at Life's End

If each person were his own judge, and had to judge himself for all of his actions, after watching a movie of his entire life, what sentence would each one give himself? I ask this question because I have had the opportunity to know and hear the testimonies of five people who were clinically dead, but were then revived. The sequences of the events following the separation of the spirit from the body vary in their nuances, but they also all had a similar event: as soon as they perceived that they were leaving their bodies, in a fraction of seconds, as if they were watching a movie, they relived their entire lives.

Those who had lived a normal life, in the fear of God, felt an indescribable joy when their spirits left their bodies. After the movie of their lives was shown, they entered into something like a tunnel, with a brilliant light at the other end attracting them, as if they were being sucked towards it. As they drew nearer to the light, the sensation of joy increased. But suddenly, as if something were sucking them back, they saw themselves returning to their bodies, and maintained the feeling of indescribable and supernatural peace and joy.

However, those who had not lived a life of righteousness and in the fear of God, who had committed injustices and had neglected the laws of God, began to feel a sensation of oppression when they saw the movie. And when they entered into the tunnel, they, too, saw a light, but instead of going towards it, they felt themselves being sucked downwards, away from it. This terrible and frightening experience only ceased when they returned to their bodies, still with a horrible sensation of anguish and oppression.

One person who has such a testimony was a member of a church, had been baptized, and led a life of devotion to God. Even so, when he left his body, he experienced a terrible sensation of being sucked down into the earth. He cried out in the darkness, "God! I belong to church! I have been baptized!" He cried out again, with all his strength, but there was no answer. Suddenly he found himself at the bottom of the pit, and saw the door of hell. He felt intense heat in his face. A creature came and took him by the arm, to take him into hell.

Then he heard a voice from heaven, as if it were a voice of a man, but he did not understand what was said, as it was in another language. At this moment the place shook as if it were an earthquake, and the creature let go of his arm. He felt a strong suction pulling him up from his back, away from hell. As he went he prayed, "Father, I come to you in the name of the Lord Jesus! I repent of my sins, and I beg you to forgive me!" When he arrived at the mouth of the pit, he felt a fresh breeze, and emerged head first.

At this moment he saw himself returning to his body, and his physical voice returned, continuing the prayer in a loud voice, so that many people within dozens of yards from his hospital bed, as he was later told, could hear. Then he felt a great peace, as if a tremendous weight had been removed from his chest. This experience was shared by the famous American writer, Kenneth E. Hagin, in his book, *The Name of Jesus*.

What most called my attention in these testimonies is the fact that after returning to life, all of these people began giving God preeminence in their lives, and lived uncommonly happy lives, anxiously awaiting the moment in which they would re-live that extraordinary experience, now with the certainty that death is merely a passing into something better (for those who have had a real experience with Jesus). All of these people are dedicated to the cause of God, and have been living testimonies of the message of salvation and redemption.

There are those who consider all that they do in life to be perfectly normal, even the acts of injustice and cruelty, and think that the day of their death will be the end. Therefore they care little about whether or not their actions will be harmful to others, and they are indifferent and uncaring as to what awaits them at the end of life.

As one involved in human relations, I observe what happens in the lives of many people. I can affirm, with absolute certainty that everything that a person does will, sooner or later, reflect in his personal life.

One of the things that take away a person's peace is that which is reflected in his sub conscience. Man lies, deceives, slanders, steals, betrays, and otherwise hurts other people, and thinks that no one will accuse him. His first accuser is his own spirit, which was made in the image and likeness of God. It is the spirit within us that struggles to guide the body to practice that which is good, right, and just. It is the spirit that makes our conscience weighs heavy. Existential crisis and oppression generally arise as consequences of a person's own actions.

After I begin living in accordance with the Word of God, seeking to faithfully follow its teachings, and radically changing my way of thinking and acting, honestly and correctly fulfilling all of my social and personal obligations, I never again had problems with my conscience, which has resulted in the great inner peace that I enjoy.

The more knowledge I gain in the areas of sociology, philosophy, and psychology, the more I am convinced that the Gospel of Jesus Christ is the only truth and rule of faith, is practical for this life, and the only way to find true inner peace.

I keep up with world events, and compare them to what is written in the Holy Bible. Even though the Bible says that one day every person will find themselves before God's throne of judgment, and will be judged for all that they have done, many people do not believe in the existence of heaven, much less hell. The Bible, however, is emphatic about this subject, and discusses it clearly, even citing examples.

What can we say about these facts that I mentioned, of two people who had died, who were doctors, and had already been declared legally dead? Those who do not believe in life after death should analyze the facts, and pause to meditate seriously on the subject.

Some time ago the media reported on a bank robbery that shocked the public sensitivity. During the robbery, one of the thieves became irritated because of the loud cries of a baby, and so he shot the baby through the head, also hitting the mother in the heart. Both died instantly. Then the thief was attacked by a security guard, and was killed in the site. Could it be that after having committed such a cruel and atrocious act, that all was over for that thief upon his death?

Daily we hear news reports about injustices committed by people who humiliate, hurt, and kill others out of greed, pride, or selfishness. Is it possible that those who enjoy the practice of evil and injustice will never be punished? They just die, and that's it? In light of these facts, and of the reality that we see each day in this world, I ask: "Isn't it just that the unrighteous pay for their unrighteous acts, and that those who live in righteousness also receive their reward? What reward is for the good and the evil? (The answer is in the Bible, in Matthew 13:47-50.)

Of all existing thoughts and philosophies, the only one that deals logically with these questions is the Holy Bible; "*Because all of us will appear before the judgment seat of Christ, so that each one will receive according to* the good or evil he has done in the body." (2 Corinthians 5:10.) In Romans 14:10-12 it is written, "...for all will appear before the judgment seat of God... thus each of us will give account of himself to God."

I hope that each one will examine his own conscience, and determine what his personal sentence will be at the end of life. It is my desire that each find his way, not only to a better and healthier life, a long-lasting youth, and a pleasant and peaceful old age, but most importantly, that he can live with the hope of a peaceful death, based on the certainty of the promise that the Lord Jesus made upon ascending into heaven:

"Do not let your hearts be troubled. Trust in God; trust also in me. In my Father's house are many rooms; if it were not so, I would have told you. I am going there to prepare a place for you. And if I go and prepare a place for you, I will come back and take you to be with me that you also may be where I am. You know the way to the place where I am going. Thomas said to him: "Lord, we don't know where you are going, so how can we know the way?" Jesus answered: "I am the way and the truth and the life. NO ONE COMES TO THE FATHER EXCEPT THROUGH ME" (John 14:1-6).

Commentaries

Dr. **Artenio Olivio Richter**
Aesthetician and Rejuvenatory

This work surprised me by the lightness and simplicity with which it deals with aspects of human health, which have been so greatly complicated by the multiplicity of subjects, specializations, and formulas. Man seeks the ideal of living well outside of himself and to the ends of the universe, when in reality the ideal is very near, inside himself. But he cannot see it, as it is obscured by the array of attractive options offered by life.

Thus man, in modern life, seeks to prolong life by complicated methods and formulas, always far away from himself, while Godoy shows us, through his practical experiences, that this dilatation is within us, through man's returning to himself, loving and respecting himself, nature, and the laws of the Creator, in order to live a longer and healthier life.

Man, inebriated and insane in the search for money, power, pleasures, and vices, falls into prostitution, drugs, alcohol, and gluttony. Our modern-day lifestyle leads us far from our inner self, thus cutting us off from the ideal and the purpose for which we were created. As a result, the duration and quality of life decreases.

Doctors warn: It is necessary to avoid or eliminate the causes of sicknesses. New techniques are presented, new resources are created, science progresses, but man ever increasingly suffers from sickness, for he has no time to stop, think, and listen. He prefers to be a tattered human being, always dragging behind and suffering; in short, he wants to be sick and old.

Dr. **Luiz Americo Limberti Nogueira**
Digestive System Specialist

With simplicity and perseverance, Tadeu Godoy shares his personal experience based on concepts of health that are not always easy to follow. I had the privilege of accompanying the course of struggles, revisions, and more revisions, that Tadeu had to face up until the finalization of this book, and I am sure that he reached his objective.

Very different from being a manual for perfect health, the work of Tadeu Godoy recuperates the good habits and customs so largely forgotten in our day. It also exhorts us to preserve our life as it was originally given to us by the Creator, and reminds us that the answer is in the observance of God's laws.

Dr. **Adelmo Almeida de Oliveira**
Cardiologist

During all the years of my professional medical career, I do not remember any other patient of Tadeu's age, who has undergone complete checkups with me (electro-cardiogram, blood pressure, Triglycerides, Cholesterol, Cholesterol LDL, glycoside, uric acid, and others), and who obtained the result of "excellent hemo-dynamic conditions." Besides this, he has been able to maintain the same physical characteristics of when he was 25 – a full head of hair, weight in proportion to his height (1.7 meters, 65 kilos), and firm muscles, which give him the appearance of someone 20 years his junior.

As a medical specialist, based on the personal experience of this patient, I can affirm that it is possible to prolong youthfulness and pass middle age with perfect health, and with the same vitality and energy of youth.

Dr. **Belmiro Targa**
Pediatrician

Tadeu's experience shows us that it is possible, in our days, to live a balanced life with good physical, mental, and spiritual development.

This book is the story of a friend who, thanks to his will, understanding, and great interest in human health, leads a healthy life in every aspect. Despite the fact that he has passed middle age, he still has the basic characteristics of his youth, which is something that everyone desires.

Dra. **Natalia A. L. Zambrano Barnes**
General Practitioner and Obstetrician

The day-to-day experiences that I face as a medical professional have shown me that a good part of the physical ailments that affect the health of humanity are reflexes of problems of a psychic and spiritual nature.

Therefore I am often uncomfortable treating certain patients using clinical resources to heal a physical illness when I know that it is of a psychic or spiritual origin.

I agreed to support Godoy's work because his book can be very helpful in the prevention of disease. Besides diverse orientations, it contains self-help messages and can be used as an important guide for a truly healthy life, both in the spiritual and physical realm.

About the Author

From the city of Imbituba, in the state of Santa Catarina, Tadeu Godoy was born on May 1, 1945. Besides being a writer, he is a political essayist with dozens of published articles. He is also a poet and musical composer. As a poet he published *Poetic Anthology of Brazilian Cities 1991,* which classified in the national contest promoted by Shogun do Rio de Janeiro Publishers. As a musical composer he has had compositions classify in diverse popular and sacred music festivals.

He began his experience in the area of medicine and health at age 13, when he worked behind the counter and as a nursing assistant in a drugstore. His interest in knowing about sicknesses was so great that he would spend his free time reading the descriptions and pamphlets that came with the medicines.

Due to this great interest and dedication to his work, he accumulated experience in a very short period, and was soon sought after. He was invited to work as an assistant in the clinic of Dr. Iran Iared Lopes, and also, at that time, took a nursing course. He worked as a nursing assistant until age 23, when circumstances forced him to opt for another profession. He worked in this new role, in the area of food, for 20 years, and had the opportunity to increase his knowledge of nutrition.

Though he worked in a different area, he never lost his interest in medicine and health, nutrition and youthfulness. Therefore, in order to learn more about health, he became a dedicated student, collected literature on the subject, and became knowledgeable in biomedical sciences.

From 1988 to 1990, while he was taking the technical course, "Preventive Health Methods" at the Richter Naturalistic Clinic, he worked as a representative and executive of international organizations of therapeutic medical products, which operate in various countries in association with medical clinics that specialize in aesthetics, nutrition, vitality, and youth preservation.

In order to perform his functions in this area, besides the aforementioned courses and training, and his general knowledge in the area of health (which earned him an honor of merit from one of the companies represented), he needed to take several different courses and attend lectures and seminars on medicine and health, given by the following specialists:

Artenio Olívio Richter (Nutrition, Aesthetics and Rejuvenation), João Batista de Oliveira (Rheumatology) Adelmo Almeida de Oliveira (Cardiology), Luiz Américo Limberti Nogueira (Gastrointestinal Tract), Natália A. L. Zambrano Barnes (General Practitioner, Gynecology and Obstetrics), Arthur Bellenzani Neto (Physiotherapy), Franz Salces Ruiz (Nutritional Engineering - PhD), Sideval Alves da Silva (Psychology), Carlos Dourado (Psychotherapy and Dynamics of Personal and Social Relations) and Professor Eliezer Pereira de Barros (Philosophy, Theology and Psychoanalysis).

Though he always desired to go to medical school, his life circumstances did not permit it. From 2002 to 2006 he worked once again in the area of health, and participated in various lectures and seminars in order to increase his knowledge, in the areas of personal training, psychotherapy of personal relationships, and treatments using the application of phyto-therapeutic products derived from medicinal plants.

In this work Tadeu Godoy shares his personal experience, including opinions of specialists and the results of diverse studies and research done on the factors that contribute towards accelerating or retarding the biological process of aging. His opinions are confirmed by the doctors and specialists listed on the Acknowledgment page.